Management Principles for Health Professionals

Joan Gratto Liebler, M.P.A., R.R.A.
Temple University

Ruth Ellen Levine, Ed.D., O.T.R.
Thomas Jefferson University

Hyman Leo Dervitz, M.A., R.P.T.
Temple University

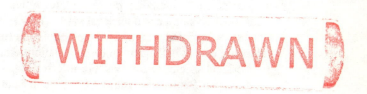

AN ASPEN PUBLICATION®
Aspen Publishers, Inc.
Rockville, Maryland
Royal Tunbridge Wells
1984

Library of Congress Cataloging in Publication Data

Liebler, Joan Gratto.
Management principles for health professionals

"An Aspen publication."
Includes bibliographies and index.
1. Health services administration. 2. Management. I. Levine,
Ruth Ellen. II. Dervitz, Hyman Leo. III. Title. [DNLM:
1. Health facilities—Organization and administration.
2. Health occupations. 3. Health services—Organization
and administration. 4. Organization and administration.
WX 150 L716m]
RA393.L53   1984   362.1'068   83-15664
ISBN: 0-89443-948-0

Publisher: John Marozsan
Editor-in-Chief: Michael Brown
Executive Managing Editor: Margot Raphael
Editorial Services: Martha Sasser
Printing and Manufacturing: Debbie Collins

Library of Congress Catalog Card Number: 83-15664
ISBN: 0-89443-948-0

Printed in the United States of America

Table of Contents

iii

Preface

This book is intended for use by health care personnel who participate in the classic functions of a manager—planning, organizing, decision making, staffing, leading or directing, communicating, and motivating—yet have not had extensive management training. Health care practitioners may exercise these functions on a continuing basis because they are department heads or unit supervisors, or they may participate in only a few of these traditional functions. In any case, a knowledge of management theory is an essential element in professional training, as no one function is carried out independently of the others. In this book, emphasis is placed on definitions of terms, clarifications of concepts, and, in some cases, highly detailed explanations. Examples are drawn from the health care setting.

Every author must decide what material to include and at what level of detail. Samuel Johnson observed that "a man will turn over half a library to make one book." We have been guided by experience gained in the classroom and in many continuing education workshops for health care practitioners. Three basic objectives determined the final selection and development of material:

1. Acquaint the health care practitioner with management concepts essential to the understanding of the organizational environment within which the functions of the manager are performed. Some material challenges assumptions about such concepts as power, authority, influence, and leadership. Some of the discussion focuses on relatively new concepts, such as the systems approach, input-output analysis, and networking. Practitioners must not be afraid of such concepts; indeed, they should guard against "being the last to know."

2. Present a base for further study of management concepts. Therefore, the classic literature in the field is cited, major theorists noted, and

terms defined, especially where there is a divergence of opinion in management literature. We all stand on the shoulders of the management "giants" who paved the way in the field; a return to original sources is encouraged.

3. Provide sufficient detail in selected areas to enable the practitioner to apply the concepts in day-to-day situations. Several tools of planning and control, such as the PERT network, management by objectives, work sampling techniques, the flow chart, and the flow process chart, are explained in detail.

We have attempted to provide enough information to make it possible for the reader to use these tools with ease at their basic level. It is the authors' hope that the reader will turn to more advanced applications as a result.

Joan Gratto Liebler
Ruth Ellen Levine
Hyman Leo Dervitz

Part I

Selected Management Functions

Chapter 1

Introduction to Management

CHAPTER OBJECTIVES

1. Define management.
2. Differentiate between management as an art and management as a science.
3. Identify the basic functions of the manager.
4. Identify the major phases in management history.

Management has been defined as the process of getting things done through and with people. It is the planning and directing of effort, the organizing and employing of resources (both human and material), to accomplish some predetermined objective. Within the overall concept of management, the function of administration can be identified. The practical execution of the plans and decisions on a day-to-day basis requires specific administrative activities that managers may assign to executive officers or administrators. Managers may find that their role includes specifically administrative activities in addition to overall management. The workday of a typical department head in a health care institution contains a mix of broad-based managerial functions and detailed administrative actions.

MANAGEMENT: AN ART OR A SCIENCE?

Especially since the turn of the century, management's scientific aspects have been emphasized. The scientific nature of management is reflected in the fact that it is based on a more or less codified body of knowledge consisting of theories and principles that are subject to study and further experimentation. Yet, management as a science lacks the distinct characteristics of an exact discipline, such as chemistry or mathematics.

The many variables associated with the human element make management as much an art as a science. Even with complex analytical tools for decision making, such as probability studies, stochastic (random) simulation, and similar mathematical elements, the manager must rely on intuition and experience in assessing such factors as timing and tactics for persuasion.

FUNCTIONS OF THE MANAGER

A manager's functions can be considered a circle of action in which each component leads to the next. Although the functions can be identified as separate sets of actions for purposes of analysis, the manager in actual practice carries out these activities in a complex, unified manner within the total process of managing. Other individuals in the organization carry out some of these activities, either periodically or routinely, but the manager is assigned these specific activities in their entirety, as a continuing set of functions. When these processes become routine, the role of manager emerges. The traditional functions of a manager were identified by Gulick and Urwick,[1] who reflected the earlier work of Henri Fayol.[2] Chester Barnard brought together the significant underlying premises about the role of the manager in his classic work, *The Functions of the Executive*.[3]

Classic Management Functions

Management functions typically include

- planning: the selection of objectives, the establishment of goals, the factual determination of the existing situation and the desired future state.
- decision making: a part of the planning process in that a commitment to one of several alternatives (decision) must be made. Others may assist in planning, but decision making is the privilege and burden of managers. Decision making includes the development of alternatives, conscious choice, and commitment.
- organizing: the design of a pattern of roles and relationships that contribute to the goal. Roles are assigned, authority and responsibility are determined, and provision is made for coordination. Organizing typically involves the development of the organization chart, job descriptions, and statements of workflow.
- staffing: the determination of personnel needs and the selection, orientation, training, and continuing evaluation of the individuals who hold the required positions identified in the organizing process.

- directing or actuating: the provision of guidance and leadership so that the work performed is goal-oriented. It is the exercise of the manager's influence, the process of teaching, coaching, and motivating workers.

- controlling: the determination of what is being accomplished, the assessment of performance as it relates to the accomplishment of the organizational goal, and the initiation of corrective action.

Figure 1–1 summarizes the classic functions of the manager and their relationship to each other. In addition, managers must continually establish and maintain internal and external organizational relationships to achieve an effective working rapport. They must monitor the organization's environment to anticipate change and bring about the adaptive responses required for the institution's survival.

At different phases in the life of the organization, one or another management function may be dominant. In the early stages of organizational development, for example, planning is the manager's primary function. When the organization is mature, however, controlling functions are emphasized.

Figure 1–1 Interrelationship of Management Functions

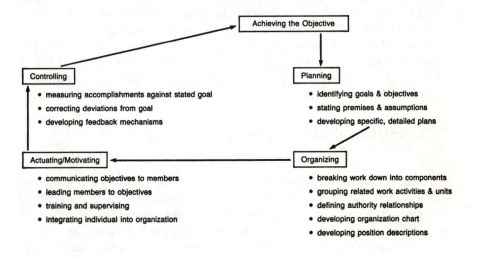

The Health Care Practitioner as Manager

In the specialized environment of a health care institution, qualified professional practitioners may assume the role of unit supervisors, project managers, and department heads or chiefs of service in their distinct disciplines. The role may emerge gradually as the number of patients increases, as the variety of services expands, and as specialization occurs within a profession. A physical therapy staff specialist, for example, may develop a successful program for patients with spinal cord injury; as the practitioner most directly involved in the work, this individual may be given full administrative responsibility for that unit. The role of manager begins to emerge: budget projections to be made, job descriptions to be updated and refined, staffing pattern to be reassessed and expanded.

An occupational therapist may find that a small program in home care flourishes and is subsequently made into a specialized unit. Again, this credentialed practitioner in a health care profession assumes the managerial role. The medical technologist who participates in the development of a nuclear medicine unit or the dietitian who develops a nutrition counseling program for use in outpatient clinics may also find themselves in this position.

The role of the professional health care practitioner as manager is reinforced further by the various legal, regulatory, and accrediting agencies that often require chiefs of service or department heads to be qualified practitioners in their distinct disciplines. The role of manager then becomes a predictable part of the health care practitioner's tenure in an institution. Table 1–1 shows how activities in a typical workday of a department head in a health care institution reflect the functions of a manager in their classic form.

THE HISTORY OF MANAGEMENT

An organization is shaped by past practices. By studying the history of management, managers can become aware of the major areas that have been emphasized during the various periods of the organization's life. As health care organizations assume more and more features of business enterprises (rather than philanthropic services), health care managers may identify certain features that are adaptations of management practices in business and industry, such as the application of industrial engineering techniques, incentive wages and bonuses, and emphasis on human relations.

Table 1-1 The Chief of Service as Manager: Examples of Daily Activities

Activity	Management Function Reflected
Readjust staffing pattern for the day because of employee absenteeism	Staffing
Review cases with staff, encouraging staff members to assume greater responsibility	Controlling Planning Leading/motivating/actuating
Counsel employee with habitual lateness problem	Controlling Leading/motivating/actuating
Present departmental quality assurance plan for approval of Risk Management/Quality Assurance Committee	Planning Leadership

A knowledge of the history of management provides a framework within which contemporary managerial problems may be reviewed. Modern managers benefit from the experiences of their predecessors. They may assess current problems and plan solutions by using theory that has been developed and tested over time. Contemporary executives may take from past approaches the elements that have been proved successful and seek to integrate them into a unified system of modern management practice.

In an examination of the phases in management history, it must be remembered that history is not completely linear and that any period in history involves a dynamic interplay of components that cannot be separated into distinct elements. The analysis of selected processes of the various historical periods tends to obscure the fact that each period is part of a continuum of events. The specific features of management history phases given here are intended to exemplify the predominant emphasis of the period, and are only highlights of the complete historical period. The second caution is that of dating the various periods. The dates given here for the various periods of management history are intended as guides. There is no precise day and year when one school of thought or predominant approach began or ended. As with any study of history, the dates suggest approximate periods when the particular practices were developed and applied with sufficient regularity as to constitute a school of management thought or a predominant approach.

Scientific Management

The work of Frederick Taylor (1865-1915) is the commonly accepted basis of scientific management. Taylor started as a day laborer in a steel mill, advanced to foreman, and experienced the struggles of middle management as the workers resisted top executives' efforts to achieve more productivity. He faced the basic question: What is a fair day's work? With Carl G. L. Barth (1860–1939) and Henry L. Gantt (1861–1919), Taylor made a scientific study of workers, machines, and the workplace. These pioneers originated the modern industrial practices of standardization of parts, uniformity of work methods, and the assembly line.

Frank Gilbreth (1868–1924) and Lillian Gilbreth (1878–1972) developed a class of fundamental motions, starting with the *therblig* (a term derived from their own name) as the most basic elemental motion. Lillian Gilbreth may be of particular interest to occupational therapists, since much of her later work concerned the efficiency of physically handicapped women in the management of their homes. The term *scientific management* became an accepted, codified concept as a result of a famous case on railroad rate structures heard by the Interstate Commerce Commission. Louis D. Brandeis, later Supreme Court Justice Brandeis, argued against rate increases by citing the probable effects of the application of "scientific management."[4] The concept emerged as the predominant approach to management during this era.

The Behavioralists and the Human Relations Approach

Although the major figures in the development of scientific management emphasized the work rather than the worker, concern for the latter was apparent. Lillian Gilbreth, for example, was a psychologist and tended to stress the needs of the employee. Frank Gilbreth developed a model promotion plan that emphasized regular meetings between the employee and the individual responsible for evaluating the work.

Unlike those who adhered to the scientific management approach, who considered the worker only secondarily, behavioralists focused primarily on the worker. The application of the behavioral sciences to worker productivity and interaction was exemplified in the Hawthorne Experiments conducted by Elton Mayo and F. J. Roethlisberger at Western Electric's Hawthorne Works. Through these studies, the importance of the informal group and the social and motivational needs of workers were recognized. The behavioral science and the human relations approaches may be linked because both emphasize the worker's social and psychological needs, stressing group dynamics, psychology, and sociology. Theorists associated with these approaches include Douglas MacGregor, Rensis Likert, and Chris Argyris.

Structuralism

Since work is done within specific organizational patterns and since the worker-superior roles imply authority relationships, the structure or framework within which these patterns and relationships occur has been studied. Structuralism is based on Max Weber's theory of bureaucracy or formal organization. Robert K. Merton, Philip Selznik, and Peter Blau, major theorists in the structuralist school of thought, gave particular attention to line and staff relationships, authority structure, the decision-making process, and the effect of organizational life on the individual worker.

The Management Process School

The special emphasis in the management process approach is on the various functions that the manager performs as a continuous process. Henri Fayol (1841–1925), a contemporary of Taylor, studied the work of the chief executive and is credited with having developed the basic principles or "laws" that are associated with management functions. His writings did not become readily available in English until 1939 when James D. Mooney and A. C. Reiley published a classification and integrated analysis of the principles of management, including Fayol's concepts.[5] Chester Barnard could be associated with this school of thought in that he explored the basic processes and functions of management, including the universality of these elements.

The Quantitative Approach/Operations Research

Problem solving and decision making with the aid of mathematical models and the use of probability and statistical inference characterize management by quantitative approach/operations research. Also called the management science school, this approach includes the various quantitative approaches to executive processes and is characterized by an interdisciplinary systems approach. The urgency of the problems in World War II and in the space program speeded the development of mathematical models and computer technology for problem solving and decision making.

THE SYSTEMS APPROACH

Each school of management thought tends to emphasize one major feature of an organization:

1. Scientific management focuses on work.

2. Human relations and behavioralism stress the worker and the worker-manager relationship.
3. Structuralism emphasizes organizational design.
4. Management process theory focuses on the functions of the manager.
5. Management science theory adds computer technology to the scientific method.

The search for a management method that takes into account each of these essential features led to the systems approach. This focuses on the organization as a whole, its internal and external components, the people in the organization, the work processes, and the overall organizational environment.

Historical Development of the Systems Model

The systems model is generally accepted in the area of computer technology, but its use need not be limited to such an application; at its origin, it was not so restricted. A more flexible use of this approach provides the manager with a framework within which the internal and external organizational factors can be visualized. The systems approach to management emphasizes the total environment of the organization. The cycle in input, transformation to output, and renewed input can be identified for the organization or for any of its divisions. The changes in organizational environment can be assessed continually in a structured manner to determine the impact of change.

Management theorists turned to biologists and other scientists to develop the idea of the organization as a total system. With this ecological approach, a change in any one aspect of the environment is believed to have an effect on the other components of the organization. The specifics are analyzed, but always in terms of the whole. The institution is considered an entity that "lives" in a specific environment and has essential parts that are interdependent.

General systems theory as a concept was introduced and defined by Ludwig von Bertalanffy, a biologist, in 1951.[6] His terminology is the foundation for the basic concepts of the general systems theory.[7] Kenneth E. Boulding developed a hierarchy of systems to help bridge the gap between theoretical and empirical systems knowledge. He noted that the general systems approach furnished a framework or skeleton for all science, but that each discipline, including management science, must apply the model, add the flesh and blood of its own subject matter, and develop this analytical model further. Included in Boulding's hierarchy of systems is the concept of the open system and the idea of the social organization with role sets.[8]

Many contemporary studies of various aspects of organizations are based on the systems model. Areas of specific application include

- cybernetics: the science of communication and control[9]

- data-processing systems: concern with the flow of information, usually by means of computer technology

- rhochrematics: the science of managing material flow, including production and marketing, transporting, processing, handling, storing and distributing goods[10]

- network analysis: the process of planning and scheduling such as PERT networks and the critical path method

- administrative systems: the planned approach to activities necessary to attain desired objectives

Basic Systems Concepts and Definitions

A system may be defined as an assemblage or combination of things or parts forming a complex or unitary whole, a set of interacting units. The essential focus of the systems approach is the relationship and interdependence of the parts. The systems approach moves beyond structure or function (e.g., organization charts, departmentation) to emphasize the flow of information, the work, the inputs, and the outputs. Systems add horizontal relationships to the vertical relationships contained in traditional organizational theory.

The systems model is made up of four basic components: (1) inputs, (2) throughputs or processes, (3) outputs, and (4) feedback (Figure 1–2). The overall environment also must be considered.

The Nature of Inputs

Inputs are elements the system must accept because they are imposed by outside forces. The many constraints on organizational processes, such as government regulation and economic factors, are typical inputs imposed by outside groups. Certain inputs are needed in order to achieve the organizational goal; for example, the inputs often are the raw material that is processed to produce some object or service. The concept of input may be

Figure 1–2 Basic Systems Model

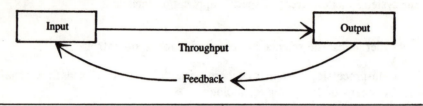

expanded to include the demands made on the system, such as deadlines, priorities, or conflicting pressures. Good will toward the organization, general support, or the lack of these also may be included as inputs.

A systematic review of inputs for a health care organization or one of its departments could include

- characteristics of clients: average length of stay, diagnostic categories, payment status
- legal and accrediting agency requirements: federal conditions of participation for Medicare programs, institutional licensure, and licensure or certification of health care practitioners
- federal and state laws concerning employers: collective bargaining legislation, the Occupational Safety and Health Act, Workers' Compensation, Civil Rights Act
- multiple goals: patient care, teaching, research

The Nature of Outputs

Outputs are the goods and services that the organization (or subdivision or unit) must produce. These outputs may be routine, frequent, predictable, and somewhat easy to identify. The stated purpose of the organization usually contains information on its basic, obvious outputs. For example, a fire department provides fire protection, a hospital offers patient care, a department store sells goods, a factory produces goods, and an airline supplies transportation. Managers control routine and predictable outputs through proper planning.

Other necessary outputs are infrequent, but predictable. By careful analysis of organizational data over a relatively long time period, these infrequent outputs can usually be identified. For example, hospitals or programs are re-accredited periodically, and plans can be made for the re-accreditation process because it is predictable. An organization that is tied directly to political sponsorship could take the cycle of presidential and congressional elections into account. Again, proper planning through identification and anticipation of such special periodic demands on the system leads to greater control and, consequently, stability.

Most managers face a third category: the nonpredictable outputs for which they can and must plan. Certain demands on the system are made with sufficient regularity that, although the exact number and time cannot be calculated, estimates can be made. This is an essential aspect of proper planning and controlling. In an outpatient clinic, for example, the number of walk-in and/or emergency patients is not predictable. In order to plan for these relatively random demands on the system, the manager studies the pattern of walk-in patients, their times of arrival, and the purposes of their visits. Some patient education would probably be done to help clients take advantage of orderly scheduling. Staffing patterns would be adjusted to meet the anticipated needs. The planning is designed to shift the nonpredictable to the predictable as far as possible. Other examples of nonpredictable outputs for which plans can be developed include telephone calls, employee turnover rates, and even activities required by certain kinds of disasters, such as seasonal tornadoes or hurricanes, or seasonal changes in number and types of clients (e.g., in a resort area).

Some outputs are unexpected, such as those that become necessary because of natural disasters or sudden economic chaos. Even in these instances, managers can anticipate and plan for Armageddon in any of its symbolic or real forms. Disaster planning, for example, is a required part of institutional health care management.

Some outputs for health care institutions are

- maintenance of accreditation and licensure status
- compliance with special federal programs concerning quality assurance or health care planning
- provision of acute care services for medical, surgical, obstetric, and pediatric patients
- provision of comprehensive mental health services for clients in a specific area

Outputs in health care institutions may be refined even further by adding specific time factors, quality factors, or other statements of expected performance:

- processing of specified laboratory tests within ten hours of receipt of specimen
- retrieval of patient medical record from permanent file within seven minutes of receipt of request

• 100 percent follow-up on all patients who fail to keep appointments

It may be useful to group outputs with the related inputs by formulating input/output statements. It should be noted, however, that not every input generates a direct output; there is no one-to-one ratio of input to output. It may be necessary to consider a cluster of inputs in relation to the output. For example, the goal (output) of retrieving the medical record of a patient who enters the walk-in clinic without an appointment and cannot be treated until the chart has been obtained may require the following considerations (inputs):

Inputs	Output
Hospital policy concerning chart availability for patients before receiving treatment	Retrieval of patient chart within seven minutes of request
Random arrival of patient and therefore of request for medical record	
Patient identification incomplete	
Incomplete or unavailable charts	
Misfiles within storage area	

Throughputs (Withinputs)

Throughputs are the structures or processes by which inputs are converted to outputs. Physical plant, workflow, methods and procedures, and hours of work are throughputs. Inputs originate in the environment of the organization; throughputs, as the term implies, are contained within the organization. Throughputs are analyzed by work sampling, work simplification, methods improvement, staffing patterns, and physical layout analysis.

Managers may be severely limited in their ability to control inputs, but the processes, structures, organizational patterns, and procedures that constitute the throughputs are normally areas of management prerogative. For example, a chief of service cannot control patient arrivals for walk-in service in a clinic; this input is imposed on the system. The policies and procedures for processing walk-in patients, however, constitute a cluster of throughputs that can be determined by the manager. The physical space allotment for a department may be imposed; the manager must accept this input, but the final and detailed physical layout of the department is under the manager's control.

In a specialized service, the control of throughputs is directly related to the manager's professional knowledge. For example, procedures for processing patient flow within a clinic are developed by the chief of service because of that person's knowledge of patient care procedures, priorities, and the interrelationships among components of the treatment plan. The policies and procedures for the release of information from patients' medical records are aspects of highly technical processes that are the domain of the professional medical record practitioner.

In some cases, elements that theoretically belong to the throughput category are considered inputs. These are elements that are imposed by the environment, i.e., the organization as a whole. Managers may not be able to exert direct control over some aspects of the work, such as physical space limitations, budget cuts, and personnel vacancies, and these elements could be listed as special inputs.

Feedback

Changes in the input mix must be anticipated. In order to respond to these changes, managers need feedback on the acceptability and adequacy of the outputs. It is through the feedback process that inputs, and even throughputs, are adjusted to produce new outputs. The communication network and control processes are the usual sources of organized feedback. Routine, orderly feedback is provided by such activities as market research and forecasting in business organizations, client surveys in service organizations, periodic accreditation surveys in health care institutions, periodic employee evaluations in work groups, and periodic testing and grading in an educational system. The management by objectives process, short interval scheduling, and Program Evaluation Review Technique (PERT) networks constitute specific management tools of planning and controlling that include structured, factual feedback.

If there is an absence of planned feedback, if the communication process is not sufficiently developed to permit safe and acceptable avenues for feedback, or if the feedback is ignored, feedback will occur spontaneously. In this case, it tends to take a negative form, such as a client outburst of anger, a precipitous lawsuit, a riot, a wildcat strike, a consumer boycott, or an epidemic. Spontaneous feedback could take a positive form, of course, such as the acclamation of a hero or leader after a crisis or an unsolicited letter of satisfaction from a client.

Some feedback is tacit, and the manager may assume that, since there is no overt evidence to the contrary, all outputs are fine. The danger in such an assumption is that problems and difficulties may not come to light until a crisis occurs. The planning process is undermined because there are no reliable data that can be used to assess the impact of change and to implement the necessary adjustments.

Closed Systems vs. Open Systems

Systems may be classified as either closed or open. An ideal closed system is complete within itself. No new inputs are received, and there is no change in the components; there is no output of energy in any of its forms, e.g., information or material. Few, if any, response or adaptation systems are needed because such a system is isolated from external forces in its environment and internal change is self-adjusting. Examples of closed systems are a chemical reaction taking place in a sealed, insulated container; a sealed terrarium; and a thermostat. In certain approaches to organizational theory, organizations have been viewed as closed systems, i.e., the emphasis has been placed on the study of functions and structure within the organization, without consideration of its environment and the consequent effect of environmental change on its processes.

An open system is in a constant state of flux. Inputs are received and outputs produced. There is input and output of both matter and energy, continual adaptation to the environment, and, usually, an increase of order and complexity with differentiation of parts over time.

An open system constantly seeks internal balance, or homeostasis, by means of an adjustive function of stimulus-response. A change in organizational environment (stimulus) makes it necessary to take some action (response) to maintain this balance. Notterman and Trumbull, using a laboratory model, noted three processes necessary for a system to maintain this self-regulating cycle:[11]

1. detection. For regulation to take place, the disparity between the disturbed and normal (or desired) state must be detectable by the organism. Obviously, if the organism cannot sense a disturbance (perceptually or physiologically), measures cannot be taken for its correction. Equally apparent is the fact that individuals vary in both the quality and quantity of information they require in order to detect a disturbance.

2. identification. The disparity must also be identified. Corrective action cannot be specific unless a given disturbance is successfully discriminated from other possible disturbances. Here again, individual differences in the form and quantity of information necessary for identification undoubtedly exist.

3. response availability. Upon detection and identification of the disturbance, the organism must be permitted by environmental, physiological, or laboratory conditions to make the correction.

Management functions of decision making, leadership, and, particularly, correction of deviation from organizational goals are necessary for the detection, identification, and proper response to changes in the organization's environment. In the open system, the adjustment to the environmental change is made through the input-output cycle and the development of appropriate feedback mechanisms. Another major management function, then, becomes the systematic monitoring of change.

All living organisms have the capacity for maximum disorder, disintegration, and death. This tendency toward disintegration is termed *entropy*. The open system is characterized by the continual striving for negative entropy *(negentropy)*. It tries to overcome disintegration by taking into itself more inputs or higher level inputs that it needs to produce the required outputs. Obvious examples of this include a bear storing body fat and changing its metabolism for winter hibernation or the human body building up immunity. In the management context, an organization may build a reserve of money or client good will against potential hard times.

Application of General Systems Theory

The systems approach enables managers to focus on the organization as a whole and to view each particular division or unit in an organization in relation to the whole. Through the systems approach, managers can cut across organizational lines to determine interrelationships in the workflow and to assess complexities in the structure and in the environment of the organization. Their attention is drawn to changes in the environment that affect the organization and its units. Managers are aided in their analysis of the organization because the input/output model frees them of personal bias toward or attachment to the existing mode of operations. Furthermore, the classic functions of a manager, which are carried out in the distinct, unique environment of a given organization, are reflected in the systems approach. Table 1-2 summarizes this interrelationship. The remainder of this presentation of management principles is developed in the context of specific functions of the manager, carried out in an overall organizational environment. Since the functions of the manager are shaped and modified by the particular organizational environment, the tools for analyzing the organization will be presented first, followed by detailed discussion of individual management functions.

Table 1–2 Relationship of Classic Management Functions and Systems Concepts

Systems Concept	Predominant Management Function
Input Analysis	
Identification of constraints	
Assessment of client characteristics	Planning
Assessment of physical space	
Budget allocation analysis	
Throughput Determination	
Development of policies, procedures, methods	Planning and controlling
Development of detailed departmental layout	
Specification of staffing pattern	Staffing
Methods of worker productivity enhancement	Controlling, leadership and motivation
Output Analysis	
Goal formulation	Planning
Statement of objectives	
Development of management by objectives plan	Planning and controlling
Feedback Mechanisms	
Development of feedback processes	Controlling, communicating, and resolving conflict
Adjustment of inputs and outputs in light of feedback	Renewing planning cycle
Adjustment of internal throughputs	

NOTES

1. Luther Gulick and Lyndall F. Urwick, eds., *Papers on the Science of Administration* (New York: Institute of Public Administration, 1937).

2. Henri Fayol, *General and Industrial Administration* (Geneva, Switzerland: International Management Institute, 1929).

3. Chester Barnard, *The Functions of the Executive* (Cambridge, MA: Harvard University Press, 1968).

4. Louis D. Brandeis, "Scientific Management and Railroads," *The Engineering Magazine,* 1911.

5. James Mooney and A.C. Reiley, *The Principles of Organization* (New York: Harper, 1939).

6. Ludwig von Bertalanffy, "General Systems Theory: A New Approach to the Unity of Science," *Human Biology* (December 1951): 303–361.

7. Ludwig von Bertalanffy, "General Systems Theory: A Critical Review," *General Systems* 7 (1962): 1–20.

8. Kenneth E. Boulding, "General Systems Theory: The Skeleton of Science," *Management Science* 2 (1956): 197–208.

9. Norbert Weiner, *The Human Use of Human Beings: Cybernetics and Society* (Garden City, NY: Doubleday Anchor, 1954).

10. Stanley H. Brewer, *Rhochrematics: A Scientific Approach to the Management of Material Flows* (Seattle, WA: University of Washington Bureau of Business Research, 1960).

11. Joseph M. Notterman and Richard Trumbull, "Notes on Self-Regulating Systems and Stress," *Behavioral Science* 4 (October 1950): 324–327.

BIBLIOGRAPHY

George, Claude S. *The History of Management Thought.* Englewood Cliffs, NJ: Prentice-Hall, Inc., 1968.

Heyel, Carl. *The Encyclopedia of Management,* 2nd ed. New York: Van Nostrand Co., 1973.

Chapter 2

Planning

CHAPTER OBJECTIVES

1. Define the management function of planning.
2. Identify the characteristics of plans.
3. Identify the participants in the planning process.
4. Indicate the constraints or boundaries on planning.
5. Identify the characteristics that make plans effective.
6. Define and differentiate among the terms *philosophy, goal, objective, functional objective, policy, procedure, method,* and *rule.*
7. Illustrate these terms through examples.

Planning is the process of making decisions in the present to bring about an outcome in the future. It involves determining appropriate goals and the means to achieve them, stating assumptions, developing premises, and reviewing alternate courses of action. It is the what-who-when-how of alternate courses of action and of possible future actions. In planning, the manager contemplates the state of affairs desired for the future.

CHARACTERISTICS OF PLANNING

Planning is the most fundamental management action and logically precedes all other management functions. Unplanned action cannot be controlled properly, because there is no basis on which to measure progress; organizing becomes meaningless and ineffective because there is no specific goal around which to mobilize resources. Decisions may be made without planning, but they will lack effectiveness unless they are related to a goal.

Planning goes beyond mere judgments, since judgments involve the assessment of a situation, but do not stipulate action to be taken. Planning includes an action to be taken, with reference to a specific goal.

In planning, the ideal state is first identified. Then the plan to achieve that ideal is modified, refined, and brought to a practical level through a variety of derived elements, such as intermediate target statements, functional objectives, and operational goals. Planning includes the decision-making process, particularly in the commitment phase. Logical planning includes commitment in terms of time and actions to be taken. There is a hierarchy in the process that includes the relationship of derived plans to the master course, the linkage of short-range and long-range plans, and the coordination of division and department or unit plans with those of the organization as a whole. Finally, planning is characterized by a cyclic process in which some or many goals and specific objectives are recyled.

In a sense, some plans are never achieved completely; they are continuous. For example, the goal of health care institutions to provide quality patient care is a continuing one that invests the many derived plans with a fundamental purpose. This goal is recycled during each planning period.

PARTICIPANTS IN PLANNING

Top-level managers set the basic tone for planning, determine overall goals for the organization, and give direction on the content of policies and similar planning documents. This is not done in isolation, but is based on information provided through the feedback cycle, through reports and special studies, and through the direct participation of personnel in each department or division.

Department heads are normally responsible for the planning process in their areas of jurisdiction. They identify overall goals and policies for their department, and they develop immediate objectives, taking into account their department's particular work constraints. In some organizations, a special planning department is created, such as a program and development division or a research and development unit.

Occasionally, clients participate in the planning process; such participation is required in some federally funded programs. In health care planning, for example, both provider and consumer membership is designated at each level of the review process. Professional associations frequently involve their members in the planning process at local, regional, state, and national levels.

The Planning Process

Since planning is intended to focus attention on objectives and to offset uncertainty, there must be a clear statement of goals. Once the goals to be attained have been established, premising must be developed, that is, the assumptions must be identified, stated, and used consistently. Premising includes an analysis of planning constraints and a statement of the anticipated environment within which the plans will unfold. In a health care organization, the premises reflect the level of care, the specific setting (e.g., outpatient clinic, inpatient unit, or home care), the specific number of beds per service, the anticipated number and kinds of specialty services or clinics, morbidity and mortality data for the outreach territory, and the availability of related services.

The department head states the premises on which departmental plans are based, e.g., the number of inpatient beds, the readmission rate, the projected length of stay, and the interrelationship of the workflow. The following is an example of specific planning premises or assumptions based on the operation of a physical therapy service:

1. Anticipated hours of operation
   a. 6 days per week
   b. 8-hour day; evening coverage for selected patients and clinics
2. Anticipated caseload
   a. Inpatients—68 per day
   b. Outpatients—15 per day
3. Diagnostic categories
   a. Hemiplegics
   b. Arthritics
   c. Amputees
   d. Fractures
   e. Sports injuries
4. Patient characteristics
   a. Adults
   b. Children
5. Level of care
   a. Acute
   b. Subacute
   c. Convalescent
   d. Chronic

Alternate approaches to reaching the desired state are developed, and the choices to be made are stated. Commitment to one of these choices constitutes the decision-making phase. Derivative plans then are formulated, and details of sequence and timing are identified. Planning includes periodic checking and review, which leads into the control process. Review and necessary revisions of plans, based on feedback, are the final steps in the cycle of planning.

PLANNING CONSTRAINTS OR BOUNDARIES

To constrain means to limit, to bind, to delineate freedom of action. Constraints in planning are factors that managers must take into account in order to make their plans feasible and realistic. Constraints, which are both internal and external, take a variety of forms. Analysis of the organizational environment by means of the clientele network, specifically the category of "controller," leads to ready identification of planning constraints. (See Chapter 15 for discussion of this concept.) The use of the input-output model also yields practical information about the constraints specific to an organization. The planning process itself imposes a constraint because of time factors. Sometimes a manager must settle for speed rather than accuracy in gathering the data needed for planning. The cost of data gathering and analysis is another constraint; if committees or special review groups are involved, the cost of their time must be noted.

The general resistance to change impedes the planning process so that standing plans take on the force of habit. Without a program for regular review of plans, they become static and rooted in tradition. Precedent becomes the rule, and the bureaucratic processes become entrenched. The phase in the life cycle of the organization also affects planning, as the degree of innovation appropriate varies with each phase.

The nature of the organization also shapes the planning process. The extent to which the organization's members participate in planning correlates with the predominant mode of authority. Highly normative organizations tend to include more member participation in their planning than do coercive ones. Ethics and values of the larger society, of the individual members, and, in health care, of the many professional organizations, help shape the goal formulation and subsequent policies and practices. When health care is seen as a right and not a privilege, there may be a greater openness to innovation and a demand for outreach programs and flexible patterns of delivery of service.

Within the organization, interdepartmental relationships may be constraints. In highly specialized organizations with many services or departments, each unit manager must consider how other departments' needs and processes are interwoven with those of the given department. Effective planning includes an assessment of such factors. The manager sometimes must accept as inputs or constraints the procedures and policies of another department.

Capital investments must also be considered. When a major commitment that involves the physical layout of the facility or some major equipment purchase has been made, the degree of flexibility in changing such processes is necessarily limited.

External factors to be considered in planning include the political climate, which varies in its openness to extensive programs in health care. The era of a Great Society approach may be replaced by an era in which an attempt is made to return health care delivery to private rather than government sponsorship, or the emphasis may shift from the federal government to the state government level. The general state of labor relations and the degree to which unionization is allowed and even mandated in an industry may be imposed on the organization. The many regulations, laws, and directives constitute another set of constraints.

In health care organizations, the many legal and accrediting requirements are specific, pervasive constraints that affect every aspect of planning. Such requirements can be developed into a reference grid for the use of the manager, since compliance with these mandates is a binding element in the overall constraint on departmental functioning.

An alternate approach to the identification of constraints in any health care planning situation is the systematic recognition of the following major factors:

1. general setting. The level and particular emphasis of care must be determined. For example, the goal of one institution may be acute care in specialized diagnostic categories; the goal of another may be the long-term care of the aged. The critical organizational relationships that stem from the general setting should be identified, e.g., the institution's degree of independence versus its adherence to corporate and affiliation agreements and contractual arrangements. Physical location may also be a constraining factor, although an earlier decision to develop the facility in a specific location may be part of the ideal plan. For example, the decision to develop a pattern of decentralized care in order to enhance the outreach program of a community mental health center will serve as a constraint on many derived plans, such as workflow and staffing patterns.

2. legal and accrediting agency mandates. Each health care institution is regulated by a federal or state agency that imposes specific requirements for the level of care and nature of services offered. For example, a hospital is licensed by the state only after it meets certain requirements; it is approved for participation in the Medicare and Medicaid programs only after it fulfills certain conditions. In addition, a hospital must comply with special regulations for medical care evaluation and health planning agency requirements for changes in bed capacity or services offered. It also must comply with malpractice insurance regulations and related risk management programs as well as fire, safety, and zoning codes, as a minimum.

3. characteristics of the clients. The general patterns of mortality and morbidity for a given population must be considered, as well as related factors such as length of inpatient stay, frequency of outpatient services, emergency unit usage, and readmission rate. Patient source of payment relates to the stability and predictability of cash flow. Specific eligibility for treatment may be another factor, as in certain community mental health/mental retardation programs, services for veterans, or programs for other specific groups.

4. practitioners and employees. The licensure laws for health care practitioners and physicians, as well as the many federal and state laws pertaining to most classes of employees, govern the utilization of staff. These include the Labor Management Relations Act (Taft-Hartley Act) the Civil Rights Act, the Age Discrimination in Employment Act, Unemployment Compensation and Workers' Compensation Acts, and the Occupational Safety and Health Act. The personnel practices mandated in the accrediting agency standards and guidelines of health agencies and professional associations also must be followed. Any contractual agreement resulting from the collective bargaining process must be taken into account. The specific bylaws and related rules and regulations for medical staff and allied health care practitioners are yet another constraint on plans involving employees and professional practitioners in any role.

CHARACTERISTICS OF EFFECTIVE PLANS

Effective plans have flexibility. Plans should have a built-in capacity to change, an adaptability. A plan could include a timetable sequence, for example, that allows extra time for unexpected events before the plan becomes off schedule.

The manager seeks to balance plans between overaim and underaim, between too idealistic and too practical or limited. Plans that are too idealistic tend to produce frustration because they cannot be attained; they may become mere mottoes. On the other hand, plans that are too modest lack motivational value, and it may be difficult to muster support for them. Clarity and vagueness must also be balanced in formulating plans. These factors help make the goals realistic. A precise goal may be a motivational tool because it provides immediate satisfaction, but there also is merit in a degree of vagueness because with some plans, especially long-range ones, it may not be possible or desirable to state goals in precise terms. Vagueness can contribute to motivation since it permits the development of detailed plans by those more directly involved in the work. Finally, vagueness can provide the necessary latitude to compromise when this is required or is a strategic action in the development of plans throughout the organization.

Types of Plans

The planning process involves a variety of plans that develop logically from the highly abstract, as in a statement of philosophy or ideal goals, to the progressively concrete, as in operational goals and procedures. Management literature on planning consistently includes the concepts of goals and objectives as central to the planning process. The terms goals and objectives frequently are used in an interchangeable manner, except in discussions of management by objectives (MBO). The MBO concept refers to specific, measurable, attainable plans for the unit, department, or organization. For the purposes of this discussion of plans, the concept of goal will be discussed in terms of overall purpose. The concept of objective will be discussed in terms of more measurable attainable plans, including unit or departmental objectives and functional objectives. Exhibit 2–1 lists the sequence of planning documents from planning state through controlling by means of operational goals.

PHILOSOPHY OR UNDERLYING PURPOSE

Individuals who share a common vision and set of values come together to create a formal organization for purposes that are consistent with and derived from their common values. The statement of philosophy or underlying purpose provides an overall frame of reference for organizational practice; it is the basis of the overall goals, objectives, policies, and derived plans. Actual practice, as delineated in policy and procedure, should not violate the organization's underlying philosophy. As new members and clients are attracted to

Exhibit 2–1 Relationship of Types of Plans

```
I.    Underlying Purpose/Overall Mission/Philosophy/Goal
         II.  Objectives
                III.  Functional Objectives
                IV.  Policies
                         V.  Procedures
                                 V.1 methods
                                 V.2 rules
                         VI.  Work Standards
                         VII.  Performance Standards
                VIII.  Training Objectives
                                 IX.  Management by Objectives
                                 X.  Operational Goals
```

the organization and as the organization grows from the gestational to the youthful stage, the statement of principles may be made more explicit. A philosophy may take one of several forms, such as a preamble, a creed, a pledge, or a statement of principle.

In addition to reflecting the values of the immediate, specific group that formed the organization, a statement of philosophy may reflect, implicitly or explicitly, the values of the larger society. To one degree or another, for example, society as a whole now accepts the burden of providing for those who need medical care. The concept of health care as a right, regardless of ability to pay, gradually emerged as an explicit value in the 1960s. Emphasis on the rights of consumers and patients emerged in a similar evolutionary pattern in the 1970s. Because free enterprise is a benchmark of the democratic way of life, a trend toward marketing and competition in health care may be noted as a feature of the 1980s.

Department managers in a health care organization are guided by several philosophical premises. These may differ from, and even be in opposition to, the managers' personal values. As members of the executive team, the managers are expected to accept these premises, however. One purpose of such practices as orientation and motivation is to foster acceptance of the underlying purpose of the organization. Typical philosophical premises in health care include

- the basic philosophy of the group that sponsors and/or controls the health care institution, e.g., federal or state government agency, religious or fraternal organization, business concern

- the American Hospital Association's guidelines on patient's rights and similar issues

- guidelines of accrediting agencies, such as the Joint Commission on the Accreditation of Hospitals (JCAH), that emphasize continuity of care, patient's rights
- guidelines, codes of ethics, and position statements of professional associations, e.g., American Physical Therapy Association, American Medical Record Association, American Occupational Therapy Association
- values of society in general, such as the current concern for privacy, equal access, employee safety, and consumer/client participation in decision making
- contemporary trends in the delivery of health care, such as the shift from inpatient acute care to outpatient, home care and community-based outreach centers; the establishment of independent practices by health professionals, e.g., nurses, who formerly provided care only under the direct supervision of physicians; the emergence of technical levels in several health professions and the acceptance of the care given by technicians

The following are excerpts from statements of philosophy. One medical record department has its philosophy stated in a preamble:

Given the basic right of patients to comprehensive, quality health care, the medical record department, as a service department, provides support and assistance within its jurisdiction to the staff and programs of this institution. A major function of this department is to facilitate continuity of patient care through the development and maintenance of the appropriate medical information systems which shall reflect all episodes of care given by the professional and technical staff in any of the components of this institution.

An educational institution adheres to the following statement of philosophy:

One of the critical elements in an effective approach to health care is the establishment of the spirit and practice of cooperative endeavor among practitioners. Recognizing this need, the Consortium for Interdisciplinary Health Studies seeks to foster the team approach to the delivery of health care.

The statement of educational philosophy of the American Medical Record Association contains the following:

Formal and informal continuing education is recognized as an essential component of professional development for health personnel. It is the task of the professional organization to assist and encourage employers and employees to participate in and support programs of continuing education.

The following is from the statement of philosophy of a physical therapy department:

> The physical therapy department as a component of the health care system is committed to providing quality patient care and community services in the most responsive and cost effective manner possible. In addition, the department will participate in research and investigative studies and provide educational programs for hospital personnel and affiliating students from the various medical and health professions.

OVERALL GOALS

The goals of the organization originate in the common vision and sense of mission embodied in the statement of purpose or the underlying philosophy. They reflect the general purpose of the organization and provide the basis for subsequent management action. As statements of long-range organizational intent and purpose, goals are the ends toward which activity is directed. In a sense, a goal is never completely achieved, but rather is a continuing, ideal state to be attained.

Goals serve as a basis for grouping organizations, e.g., educational organizations, health care institutions, and philanthropic or fraternal associations. Goals, like statements of philosophy, may be found in the organization's charter, articles of incorporation, statement of mission, or introduction to the official bylaws. Again like the statement of philosophy, the overall goals may not bear a specific label; they may be identified only through common understanding. The planning process is facilitated when the philosophy and the goals are formally stated. Derivative plans may then be developed in a consistent manner, with less risk of implementing policy and procedure that violate some otherwise implicit assumption of values.

OBJECTIVES

In the planning process, the manager makes the plans progressively more explicit. The move from the ideal, relatively intangible statements of mission and purpose or overall goal to the "real" plans is accomplished through the development of specific objectives that bring the goals to a practical, working level. Objectives are the more tangible, concrete plans, usually stated in terms of results to be achieved. The manager reviews the underlying purpose and basically answers the question: What is my unit or department to accomplish specifically in light of these overall goals?

Statements of specific objectives are continuing in nature; the work of the department must satisfy these objectives over and over again. An overall goal such as "to promote the health and well-being of the community" can be accomplished only through a series of specific objectives that are met on a continuing basis. Objectives add the dimensions of quality, time, accuracy, and priorities to goals. The objectives are specific to each unit or department, while the overall goals for an organization remain the same for all units.

Objectives may be stated in a variety of ways, and different levels of detail may be used. For example, objectives may be expressed as

- a quantifiable statement: to maintain the profit margin of 6 percent during each fiscal year by an increase in sales volume sufficient to offset increased cost.

- a qualitative statement: to make effective use of community involvement by the establishment of an advisory committee with a majority of members drawn from the active clients who live in the immediate geographical community.

- services to be offered: to provide comprehensive personal patient care services with full consideration for the elements of good medical care, e.g., accessibility, quality, continuity, and efficiency.

- a value to be supported: to ensure privacy and confidentiality in all phases of patient care interaction and documentation.

Objectives for the department as a whole may include elements essential for proper delineation of all other objectives. These may be stated as objectives for the organization and need not, therefore, be repeated in the subsequent departmental statement of objectives:

- compliance with legal, regulatory, and accrediting standards and with institutional bylaws.

- risk management factors, including accuracy. At this phase, planning is based on 100 percent accuracy.

- privacy and confidentiality in patient care transactions and documentation.

- reference to inpatient as well as outpatient/ambulatory care and other programs sponsored by the organization, such as home care or satellite clinics.

Because they are intended to give specificity to overall goals, objectives are the key to management planning. Therefore, objectives must be measurable whenever possible. They must provide for formal accountability in terms of achieving the results. Furthermore, they must be flexible so that they can be adapted to changing circumstances over time. Two additional planning concepts must be used with the statements of objectives in order to make them meaningful: the statement of functional objectives and the development of policies. These related plans are both important in fleshing out departmental objectives.

FUNCTIONAL OBJECTIVES

A functional objective is a statement that refines a general objective in terms of

- specific service to be provided
- type of output
- quantity and/or specificity of output
- frequency and/or specificity of output
- accuracy
- priorities

Some elements, such as accuracy indicators, may be defined for the department or unit as a whole. A general objective's priority may be implied by its delineation in a related functional objective.

Planning data for organizing and staffing functions may be obtained by inference from statements of objectives; for example, the functional objective statement may include the stipulation that all discharge summaries shall be typed. The workload (number of discharge summaries) may be calculated based on the number of discharges per year. A priority system for processing such summaries or a designated turnaround time for such processing provides the necessary parameters for calculating the number of workers needed to meet the objective on a continuing basis. The staffing patterns for day, evening, and night shifts may be developed, again, in a way to satisfy the priority designation and turnaround time contained in the functional objective.

The relationship of the general objective and the functional objectives that support it are clearly seen in the following example drawn from the plans for a transcription/word processing unit of a medical record department.

General Objective: The medical record department will provide a system for dictation of selected medical reports by specified health care providers and for the transcription of these reports on a routine basis.

Functional Objectives: More specifically, this system will provide for:

a) dictation services for attending medical staff, house officers and allied medical staff as defined by the medical staff bylaws.

b) transcription of reports will be done within the following time frame:

   1. discharge summaries within three working days of receipt of dictation

   2. operative reports within 24 hours of dictation

   3. consultation reports within 24 hours of dictation.

This example specifies the quantity of output, the time frame, and implicit priority through the designation of the time frame. A statement of accuracy is not included, because it is included in the objectives for the department as a whole. This accuracy statement, which may fall under the overall objective of risk management/quality control, may be expressed as follows:

The medical record department strives to carry out its responsibilities and activities within 100% accuracy; however, an acceptable level of accuracy will be established both for individual employees as well as for each subsystem of the department.

The following is an example of a general objective and functional objectives from a direct patient care service:

General Objective: The physical therapy department will provide evaluation and assessment procedures appropriate to the patient's condition as requested by the referring physician.

Functional Objectives: More specifically,

a) evaluations will be completed within two working days following receipt of the referral

b) verbal summary of findings submitted to the physicians following the completion of the evaluation

c) written summary of the evaluation noted in the patient's chart within 24 hours following the verbal report.

POLICIES

Policies are the guides to thinking and action by which managers seek to delineate the areas within which decisions will be made and subsequent action taken. Policies spell out the required, prohibited, or suggested courses of action. The limits at either end of these actions are stated, defined, or at least clearly implied. Policies predecide issues and limit actions so that situations that occur repeatedly are handled in the same way. Because policies are intended to be overall guides, their language is broad.

A balance must be found when policies are formulated. These comprehensive guides to thinking and action should be sufficiently specific to provide the user with information about the action to take, the action to be avoided, and when and how to respond; at the same time, however, they should be flexible enough to accommodate changing conditions. They should reinforce and be consistent with the overall goals and objectives. In addition, they should conform to legal and accrediting mandates, as well as to any other requirement imposed by internal or external authorities.

Wording of Policies

Policies permit and require interpretation. Language indicators, such as "whenever possible" or "as circumstances permit," are expressions typically used to give policies the flexibility needed. Policy statements in a health care institution may concern such items as definitions of categories of patients and designation of responsibility. In a medical record department, policy statements may specify such items as a standardized medical record format, internal and external distribution of copies, use of abbreviations, processing of urgent requests, and detailed delineation of those allowed to use the dictation system.

In order to decrease the sheer volume of policy statements, a glossary of terms may be developed to include such elements as a definition of patient for the institution, members of the medical and professional staff, and legal and accrediting bodies. Occasionally, a statement of rationale is included in a policy statement, but the manager should avoid excessive explanations; in general, the manager needs to couch policy directives in wording that predecides issues and permits actions.

The wording in the following examples, drawn from a variety of settings, tends to be broad and elastic, yet gives sufficient information to guide the user. The first example is a policy for tuition waiver for senior citizens:

> In recognition of their efforts over the years in support of education, the college will waive tuition for academic and continuing

education courses for senior citizens who reside in the tricounty area. All residents at least 62 years of age who are not engaged in full time gainful employment are eligible under this tuition waiver policy. This policy will be subject to annual budgeted funds.

This example provides a general sense of why the college is granting this waiver: in recognition of senior citizen support over the years. The outer limits of its applicability are noted: both academic and continuing education programs are included. A definition of senior citizen is given, and the additional eligibility factors are stated. A final parameter is included to provide flexibility should circumstances change: namely, the limitation determined by the availability of budgeted funds. With this short policy, the necessary procedures can be developed for determining eligibility, and a relatively untrained worker can make the necessary determination.

The following policy guides the user in determining eligibility for certain credit courtesies.

For business customers, the open account is available only to government agencies, recognized educational institutions, and companies with a Dun and Bradstreet rating of "good" or higher.

The limits are set by delineating the kinds of agencies, and the benchmark of a specific rating is given.

The following are typical policies for health care institutions. For employee promotion:

It is the policy of this hospital to promote from within the organization whenever qualified employees are available for vacancies. The following factors shall be considered in the selection of individual employees for promotion: length of service with the organization; above-average performance in present position; special preparation for promotion. Employees on their present job for a reasonable length of time, excluding probationary period, may request promotion during the customary period in which a job is open and posted as being available.

For admission of patients to research unit:

Since the primary purpose of this unit is research in specialized areas of medicine, the primary consideration in selecting elective patients for admission to the research unit accommodations is given to the teaching and research value of the clinical findings. The research unit offers two types of service: inpatient and outpatient. The research unit reserves the right to assign patients to either service category, depending on the characteristics of the case and facilities available at the time.

For a medical record system:

The recordkeeping system shall be a unit record and a unit numbering system. Each patient shall be assigned a unit number on the first occasion of service in any component of this health care facility and shall retain that number for all subsequent visits. Recording of information from both inpatient and outpatient services shall be contained in the same medical record.

For a physical therapy department:

The Physical Therapy Department shall be open from 8:30 A.M. to 4:30 P.M. Monday through Friday, and on weekends and holidays as required to meet patient care needs.

Sources of Policy

Department or unit managers develop the policies specific to their assigned areas, but these policies must be consistent with those originated by top-level management. Policies sometimes are implied, as in a tacit agreement to permit an afternoon coffee break. An implied policy may make it difficult to enforce some other course of action, however, if the implied policy has become standard—in spite of its lack of official approval. Policies are shaped in some instances by the effect of exceptions granted; a series of exceptions may become the basis of a new policy, or at least a revision of an existing one. Certain policies may be imposed by outside groups, such as an accrediting agency or a labor union through a negotiated contract.

PROCEDURES

A procedure is a guide to action. It is a series of related tasks, given in chronological order, that constitute the prescribed manner of performing the work. Essential information in any procedure includes the specific tasks that must be done, at what time, and/or under what circumstances they must be done, and who (job title, not name of employee) is to do them. Procedures are developed for repetitive work in order to ensure uniformity of practice, to facilitate personnel training, and to permit the development of controls and checks in the workflow. Unlike policies, which are more general, procedures are highly specific and need little, if any, interpretation.

Procedures for a specific organizational unit are developed by the manager of that unit. As with other plans, departmental procedures must be coordinated with those of related departments, as well as with those developed by higher management levels for all departments. For example, the procedures for patient transport to various specialized service units, such as nuclear medicine, physical therapy, or occupational therapy, are developed jointly by the nursing service and these related departments or services. In contrast, procedures relating to employee matters may well be dictated by top-level management for the organization as a whole with little, if any, procedural development done at the departmental or unit level.

Procedure Manual Format

The format of a procedure manual may take various forms: narrative, abbreviated narrative, and playscript. The narrative style contains a series of statements in paragraph form, with special notes or explanations in subparagraphs or in footnotes (Exhibit 2–2). The abbreviated narrative form illustrates procedures through the use of key steps and key points (Exhibits 2–3 and 2–4).

When a procedure involves several workers or departments, the playscript format may be used to advantage. Each participant in the action is identified by job title, the step is given a sequence number, a key action word or words is/are stated, and action sentences are developed for the step. The playscript format is direct and specific with its focus on "who does what and when." As each step in the procedure is analyzed and stated in terms of actor, step sequence, key action word, and action sentence, ambiguity and vagueness are avoided (Exhibit 2–5).

Leslie Matthies[1] identified the following action verbs as useful in conveying central, specific ideas for procedure statements in the playscript format:

sends	uses
shows	checks
issues	places
obtains	decides
records	receives
provides	forwards
prepares	requests

An alternate use of the playscript format stresses responsible party, step sequence, and a brief statement of action (Exhibits 2–6 and 2–7).

Exhibit 2–2 Narrative Procedure Format: Procedure for Pulling Clinic Records

Most records for clinic appointments are pulled two days in advance of the appointment date. However, there are always a few late appointments scheduled for the next day for which charts were not available when the day shift file clerks prepared records for appointments. The night file clerk is responsible for locating the records needed for these appointments. Procedures are as follows:

1. Go to admitting office to obtain late appointment slips and "due to arrive for admission" slips.
2. Pull appointment slips from DUE TO ARRIVE file in the admitting office for the next day's date.
3. Check name index for register number. (*Note*: Sometimes a patient will not have a number when the appointment is scheduled, but obtains a number between the time of scheduling the appointment and the actual appointment date.)
4. Write the number on the appointment slip if you find a card in file.
5. Write "No Number" on appointment slip if you do not find a card in file.
6. Separate the blue and the white carbon copies for the "No Number" slips and leave the blue copies in alphabetical order in the "No Number" file on the counter.

Exhibit 2–3 Abbreviated Narrative Procedure Format: Procedure for Terminal Digit Filing

Key Step	Key Points
1. Terminal digit filing system	1. Read from *right to left*, two digits at a time. EXPLANATION: Records are filed in sections by the last two digits to the right, then the middle two digits, then the last two digits to the left. Example: if the history number is 06-52-18 *find it this way:*

Look here last	Look here second	Look here first
within the 18 section	within the 18 section	18
06	52	18

The last two digits (terminals) are color coded. The colors for each digit always remain the same, and once they are learned can be used in many combinations of numbers. They help you file more accurately and quickly.

Exhibit 2–4 Abbreviated Narrative Procedure Format: Procedure for Interdepartmental Coordination

Key Step	Key Points
1. Determine patient care need.	1. Review medical care record. 2. Perform appropriate evaluation procedures. 3. Complete related medical documentation, including information needed for consultation.
2. Contact appropriate department.	1. Make verbal contact via telephone. 2. Confirm through interdepartmental request form for joint conference.

Exhibit 2–5 Playscript Format

Actor	Step Sequence	Action Words	Action Sentence
File clerk	1	Verifies identification	Check patient identification as given in patient master file: full name, date of birth, number.
File clerk	2	Records identification	Enter patient identification on medical report in appropriate section on form.

Exhibit 2–6 Alternate Playscript Format: Example 1

Responsibility	Step Sequence	Action
Patient Master File Clerk	1	Check patient identification as given in patient master file: full name, date of birth, number.
Patient Master File Clerk	2	Enter patient identification on medical report in appropriate section on form.
Terminal Digit File Clerk	3	Obtain batches of medical reports from Patient Identification section.
Terminal Digit File Clerk	4	File each medical report in specific patient record in numeric order.

Exhibit 2–7 Alternative Playscript Format: Example 2

Responsibility	Step Sequence	Action
Senior Physical Therapist	1	Receives patient referral form. Enters name, date, and time received in master file.
Senior Physical Therapist	2	Assigns patient to physical therapist for evaluation.
Staff Physical Therapist	3	Arranges treatment as scheduled for patient evaluation.
Secretary	4	Requests central transportation to deliver patient and hospital chart at designated time.

The physical format of the procedure manual is important. A procedure manual should be convenient in size, easy to read, and arranged logically. If the manual is too large or too heavy for everyday use or is difficult to read because of too many unbroken pages of type, workers tend to develop their own procedures rather than refer to the manual for the prescribed steps. The choice of a format that makes it easy to update the manual (for example, loose-leaf binder) removes a major disadvantage or limitation on the manual's use: pages of obsolete procedures.

Development of the Procedure Manual

The manager who is developing a procedure manual must first determine its purpose and audience, e.g., to train new employees or to bring about uniformity of practice among current employees. The level of detail and the number and kinds of examples depend on the purpose and the audience. Clarity, brevity, and the use of simple commands or direct language improve comprehension. Action verbs that specify actions the worker must take help to clarify the instructions. Keeping the focus of the procedure specific and its scope limited permits the manager to develop a highly detailed description of the steps to be followed. The steps are listed in logical sequence, with definitions, support examples, and illustrations.

Methods improvement is a prerequisite for efficient, effective procedure development. Flow charts and flow process charts are useful adjuncts to the procedure manual because they require logical sequencing and make it possible to reduce the backtracking and bottlenecks in the workflow.

METHODS

The way in which each step of a procedure is to be performed is a method. Methods focus on such elements as the arrangement of the work area, the use of certain forms, or the operation of specific equipment. A method describes the best way of performing a task. The manager may develop methods detail as part of the training package for employee development, leaving the procedure manual free of such detail.

RULES

One of the simplest and most direct types of plans is a rule. A continuing or repeat use plan, a rule delineates a required or prohibited course of action. The purpose of rules is to predecide issues and specify the required course of action authoritatively and officially.

Like policies, rules guide thinking and channel bahavior. Rules, however, are more precise and specific than policies and, technically, allow no discretion in their application. As a result, management must direct careful attention to the number of rules and their intent. If the management intent is to guide and direct behavior rather than require or prohibit certain actions, the rule in effect becomes a policy and should be issued as such.

Like procedures, rules guide action; unlike procedures, however, rules have no time sequence or chronology. Some rules are contained in procedures: Extinguish all smoking material before entering patient care unit. A rule may be independent of any procedure and may stand alone: No Smoking. The wording of rules is direct and specific:

- Food removed from the cafeteria must be carried in covered containers.
- Books returned to the library after 4 P.M. will be considered as returned the following day, and a late fine will be charged.
- Children under the age of 12 must be accompanied at all times by an adult who is responsible for their conduct.

NOTE

1. Leslie H. Matthies, *The Playscript Procedure* (New York: Office Publications, Inc., 1961), p. 95.

Chapter 3

Planning the Functional Environment

CHAPTER OBJECTIVES*

1. Relate the planning process to immediate and long-term functional environment needs.
2. Identify the members of the planning team.
3. Analyze the functional needs in designing a facility.
4. Discuss the three phases in the design process.
5. Understand the impact of building code regulations on programming considerations.

There is a saying that the only thing we can be sure of is that things will change. This is most certainly true in the case of health care facilities. The development of new philosophies, new methods, and new equipment, as well as a myriad of other influences, brings about rapid obsolescence of the physical environment of health care facilities, whether they be physicians' offices, clinics, rehabilitation centers, special service facilities, or full-service hospitals.

It is rare today that those associated with health care reach the end of their career without some involvement in at least one planning process for either a totally new facility or a modernization/expansion program. There are many opportunities for involvement in the exciting process of developing the health care environment; however, the level of excitement and satisfaction, both in the personal achievement and in the physical product, is a direct result of the way in which the process is administered. All too often, the health care personnel who participate in a building program have little understanding of what is really involved or what should be expected at the

---

*This chapter was prepared with the assistance of Charles N. Adams, Registered Architect.

various stages in the process. This lack of understanding may be reflected in an inadequate evaluation of needs, improper sequencing of decisions, poor communication with the design professionals, or failure to obtain adequate construction funds.

APPROACHING THE PLANNING PROCESS

The factors influencing the health care environment are complex, unique, and demanding. As such, the planning necessary to translate needs into a functionally efficient and pleasing building must be comprehensive and without prejudice. Care must be taken to avoid improper influences on the process.

One factor that frequently arises in some form is "This is the way we've always done it." People are creatures of habit and normally find security in known quantities; however, this approach does little to provide an environment that reflects the complex needs of rapidly changing health care services. Another pressure is often exerted when an individual, board, or other influential group—either through mere presence or financial control—dictates a particular route to be taken without proper consideration for all factors involved. This can have a devastating and lasting impact on both immediate and long-term successes of any project. There is a problem, also, in focusing attention on only a few specific concerns rather than on the total operation of the facility. Problems in one area perceived by some as minor can, and usually do, have a major impact on the total operation because of the interrelationships of all the functions within a health care environment. Such unrecognized effects usually have both functional and economic consequences.

It is important, certainly, to evaluate past experiences, to listen to ideas from others, and to identify specific concerns; but all this must be done in the proper perspective under a comprehensive planning process. Planning for space must be approached as a serious effort, even for "minor" alterations. Done properly, it requires considerable time and effort, but it produces rewarding results.

There are two major aspects to proper planning of facilities: (1) involve the proper people on the planning team, and (2) plan for both the long-term and for immediate needs.

THE PLANNING TEAM

In the same way that a single person cannot be expected to have the depth of expertise necessary for every aspect of patient care, neither can one person have an adequate knowledge of all the varied aspects of planning for a health care facility. It requires a team of experts from several disciplines, working together, to achieve the most satisfactory results.

The nucleus of the planning team should be formed as early as possible after the need for alterations in the functional environment has been recognized. Initially, the team should include at least the facility administrator, a board member, and an architect. Other members of the team will be required at various stages in the process and, depending on the complexity of the specific project, may include any or all of the following:

1. other representatives of the facility
   - assistant administrator
   - medical chief of staff
   - director of nursing
   - attorney
   - accountant
   - department heads

2. other design professionals
   - surveyor
   - soils engineer
   - structural engineer
   - mechanical engineer
   - electrical engineer
   - interior designer
   - landscape designer

3. special consultants
   - medical services
   - equipment
   - food service
   - laundry
   - management
   - communications
   - public relations
   - marketing
   - fund raising

In most situations, the administrator or some other representative of the facility assumes the responsibility for establishing the schedule and maintaining continuity through the planning process. When the physical facilities are being altered, however, this position is generally better served by the architect. Because of the architect's particular training and knowledge of the specific requirements at critical points in the process, the architect can help ensure an efficient coordination of the total effort. It is most unfortunate when an architect is approached only after numerous critical decisions, such as budget determinations and design solutions (that may be totally incompatible) have already been made.

The planning team must formulate and evaluate the needs, translating them into the specific physical environment to serve the intended use. Each person who participates in the planning process contributes to the ultimate success of the project. To be most effective, each person must be objective in decision making, willing to investigate alternatives, have a general understanding of the whole planning process, and have a specific knowledge of what is expected from each individual.

THE PLANNING AND BUILDING PROCESS

When faced with the prospect of a new or renovated facility, many people want to see building plans and a picture of what the building or space will look like. Such overwhelming enthusiasm, pressure for a quick solution to critical space needs (usually the result of a poor planning process in the past), or a misunderstanding of the proper planning process often leads to disastrous results. Care must be taken to ensure that adequate consideration is given to both long-range and short-range (immediate need) planning.

Long-range planning is a broad approach based on reasonable expectations for needs at some point in time beyond current needs or abilities; it provides a frame of reference against which to measure decisions regarding immediate needs. Planning for immediate needs, on the other hand, is definitive in scope, should deal with that which can be implemented within a short period of time, and should always be carried out with careful consideration for its effects on the long-range plan.

Assuming that a need has been recognized and at least the nucleus of the planning team organized, there is much planning necessary before any building plans are drawn. First, the feasibility of satisfying the need must be established within the context of both immediate capabilities and a long-range plan. At this point, preliminary investigations of such factors as existing space limitations, real versus perceived needs, site restrictions, government regulations, building code requirements, and financing potential should be made. Any obstacles that must be considered before proceeding further should be identified.

Once the project has been shown to be feasible, it is necessary to formulate a definitive functional program detailing the activity to be performed in the space(s) being planned.

Functional Programming Considerations

In the formulation of the functional program, adequate consideration must be given to all factors relative to each activity area involved. The functional program data base should always include a detailed explanation of how each activity is to be carried out within the space, who is typically involved in the activity and to what degree, and how the activity relates to the other functions within the facility. In addition, an activity may have many special requirements that will affect the design. Such factors might include the following:

- accessibility. Changes in floor levels should be minimized; where changes are necessary, ramps and/or elevators must be provided to afford easy access throughout the building. Passageways and doors must have clearances adequate for wheelchairs, stretchers, and equipment; such items that will be used in the facility must be identified. Clearances required around examination or treatment equipment must be determined, and any special considerations beyond normal barrier-free design that need to be included for servicing handicapped persons must be clarified.

- interior surfaces. Required specific characteristics of floors, walls, ceilings, doors, and cabinet work must be carefully noted. Certain types of activities require finishes that are resistant to chemicals, temperatures, or other physical abuse. Areas that need special attention concerning hygienic qualities, color selection, and thermal or acoustic control must also be identified.

- acoustics. Any equipment or activity that will either generate unusual noise levels (e.g., motors, compressors, TVs, business machines) or require a special degree of isolation from external noise for proper functioning (e.g., auditory or other monitoring equipment) must be specified.

- climate control. Factors such as temperature, humidity, odor, sanitation, air movement, and pressure must be related to each activity. The characteristics of any chemicals or other sources of fumes requiring exhaust must be specifically described. In one instance, the laboratory staff of a new facility complained when fumes of a particular chemical were not effectively removed by the exhaust system. Upon investigation, it was determined that the fumes were heavier than air and were filling the entire room before being drawn out through the ceiling-mounted exhaust grille. When a new duct was extended with a grille near the floor, the problem was eliminated. This situation could have been avoided if more complete data had been supplied to the design professionals. Unfortunately, all problems are not so easily resolved.

- plumbing. Along with defining those areas that need typical toilet and hand-washing facilities, it is also necessary to describe any special plumbing fixtures, equipment requiring plumbing connections, or special water temperature controls to be included.

- lighting. Alternative lighting methods produce a wide range of effects in color definition, glare, and distribution patterns that may or may not be acceptable for a particular activity. It is, therefore, important to identify any special or preferred lighting needs for various tasks, taking into consideration both natural and artificial light.

- electrical power. When electrical equipment is not to be specified in the construction documents, it is necessary to include information regarding power requirements and types of connections needed. Requirements for special control or outlet locations and any auxiliary systems, such as nurses' call, door security, telephone, television, and intercom, must be noted.

- furnishings and equipment. A detailed list of major furnishing and equipment requirements for each space must be made. When choices are available, preferences for built-in or portable items should be noted. Locations for oxygen and suction or other special services should also be identified.

During this stage of the planning process, the bulk of the responsibility is with the facility staff, since they are most familiar with the unique characteristics of their operational programs. Depending on the scope of the project, a medical services consultant may assist the staff in preparing this functional program. Its purpose is to furnish the architect with adequate data to begin making specific space allocations in the design process.

Phases of the Design Process

Armed with this functional data base, the architect coordinates the necessary technical disciplines, involving numerous consultants, product representatives, and other design professionals. This design process is typically divided into three phases:

1. schematic design. A diagrammatic plan is developed to reflect the departmental relationships, preliminary space allocations, circulation patterns, and other major aspects of the program. Equipment layouts are not usually detailed at this point, nor is much consideration given to the external treatment. Other planning team members must review this diagrammatic plan as thoroughly as possible to determine any program deficiencies and to ensure that the conceptual design provides a satisfactory framework for the program needs.
2. design development (preliminary design). After the schematic design has been approved, the plans are refined to include more detailed definition of spatial configurations, including wall thicknesses. Equipment layouts, window locations, any special features required, and a conceptual design of the structural and mechanical systems are also usually incorporated. More attention is directed to the building form and the exterior treatment. Proper review of both the functional program and the design solution at this phase is critical, because any changes made to the design beyond this phase will have a serious economic impact on the project.
3. construction documents. The last phase of the design effort is dedicated to preparing the documents, commonly known as working drawings and specifications, from which the project will be constructed. All aspects of the design must be completely detailed in order to ensure proper understanding of the scope of work and intent of the design. The success of the construction process depends significantly on the quality of these documents.

The design portion of the planning process is a period of intense interaction of the planning team. Each step requires clear communication among all participants if an acceptable design solution is to be achieved.

Regulations

It is the architect's responsibility to ensure that the design complies with all applicable codes; however, it is also important for the facility staff to be aware of such requirements in order to understand their impact on the design process. Depending on the type of facility under consideration, there may be constraints from local, state, and federal government agencies. The various regulations normally cover site plan development, type of construction, fire protection, energy conservation measures, space allocations, handicapped accessibility, safety features, equipment, lighting, heating and ventilating, and other miscellaneous factors.

Noncompliance with applicable code requirements results in numerous problems, among which are an inability to obtain an occupancy permit allowing use of the facility, denial of necessary operating licenses, and ineligibility for specific government or private fundings. It is necessary, also, to realize that any code provides only minimum standards and that the actual operational requirements of a particular facility may impose significantly more demanding design parameters.

Bidding and Negotiation

A reasonably firm accounting of the costs of building the project as detailed in the contract documents must be established after the design has been completed. This pricing can be used as a means of selecting a contractor for the project from among several competitive bidders, or it may serve as the basis for negotiating an agreement with a previously selected contractor. If careful attention has been given to estimating the probable construction cost at various points in each of the design phases, the detailed cost analysis by the contractors should be within acceptable limits, thus allowing the project to proceed into construction.

Construction

The onset of construction usually brings with it a renewed enthusiasm in all those who have spent much time and effort in the planning process, often wondering if they would ever see building materials being worked into shape. The architect and other design professionals continue to provide the technical assistance necessary to ensure that the construction conforms to the intent of the contract documents.

When construction is completed and the spaces are in use, a final responsibility remains for the planning team. An evaluation to determine how well the functional requirements have been met is an important part of the comprehensive planning process. Such an evaluation should occur after at least six months of full operation and should involve both the facility staff and the architect.

Chapter 4

Decision Making

CHAPTER OBJECTIVES

1. Define the management function of decision making.
2. Identify the participants in the decision-making process.
3. Evaluate a decision's importance.
4. Identify the classic steps in decision making.
5. Relate organizational constraints to decision making through identification of the barriers to rational choice.
6. Identify the bases for decision making.
7. Identify the tools for decision making.

In the planning process, the step involving the choice among alternatives is designated the decision-making phase. Decision making is choosing from among alternatives to determine the course of action. Alternatives may be limited or abundant; in any case, there must be at least two options, or there is no decision, only forced choice. Herbert Simon assigned this function a primary role; he defined decision making as the main function of a manager, the most important activity the manager performs.[1] Simon added that the best way to learn about an organization is to determine where decisions are made and by whom.[2]

PARTICIPANTS IN DECISION MAKING

The decision-making function belongs primarily to top-level management, but it involves interaction among several groups and individuals in the organization. Normally, no major decision is made by any one manager. The organizational hierarchy determines the pattern of participation in the decision-making process. Top-level managers make the pervasive, critical, non-programmed, root decisions, such as selection of organizational goals and development of major policy guidelines, although they may be assisted by technical staff advisers who develop the alternatives, based on research and analysis. Line managers may also be consulted.

The organizational structure limits the decision-making ability of all other managers in terms of authority and responsibility for specific departments or units. Such middle managers make decisions for their own units or departments within the framework set by top management rulings. In addition, because middle managers usually have some specific technical competence, they are often key participants in decisions relating to these technical areas. Top management may defer to the technical competence of individual department heads, giving them a specific charge of making final decisions in their areas of expertise. The middle manager's decision mix, then, is one of routine, recurring, decisions, along with nonrecurring, in an area of specialized technical competence. For example, the director of an occupational therapy department makes the recurring, routine decisions of vacation scheduling for department employees in accordance with overall organizational guidelines and makes nonprogrammed, critical decisions, such as equipment selection for the unit. This latter decision is made on the basis of the director's specialized knowledge as an occupational therapist.

Rank and file employees are involved in decision making in both direct and indirect ways. Collective bargaining agreements may specify areas in which employees must be consulted. Sometimes their participation is limited to ratification of the contract, but their legitimate, legal claim to participation is recognized to the degree specified in the bargaining agreement. Employees are involved in the decision-making process in a continuous, although indirect, manner; all levels of management depend on the feedback provided by workers who actually perform the day-to-day activities. This feedback process may be formalized, with employees given formal recognition as participants in planning and decision making, as in the management by objectives cycle.

Clients of an organization sometimes participate in decision making. Like employees, clients may have a legitimate claim to participation because of a legislative mandate. For example, the legislation that creates and/or funds community mental health centers or health planning agencies often requires the presence of consumers and community members on advisory councils or even governing boards. Federal and state agencies are required to hold public hearings on certain issues, which fosters client participation in decision making. Members of professional associations also participate in the decision-making process. Although primarily limited to a role of ratification of decisions presented by an elected board and/or by an appointed executive officer, members of such associations can participate more actively should a group of members wish to press a claim.

The decision-making process in health care organizations has an additional dimension in that the medical staff participates in major determinations. Neither clients nor employees in the usual sense of the term, the medical staff has a tradition of involvement in hospital governance. The dual track of authority in health care organizations brings about a special situation for the chief executive officer and for line department heads who report to the administrative officer. Through its committee structure, the medical staff becomes involved directly in the operations of some departments. In the pharmacy, for example, decisions such as the use of brand names versus generic names in drug selection cannot be made by the pharmacist alone. The pharmacy and therapeutics committee of the medical staff must make the final decision. The day-to-day operations of the medical record department are the responsibility of the medical record administrator, but the medical record committee may have as a charge, stated in the bylaws, the review of the medical record system. Although the actions of the medical staff in these areas are generally limited to suggestions rather than mandates, a limit is imposed nonetheless on the decision-making power of these managers.

Chief executive officers in a health care institution hold a role similar to that of professional managers or hired administrators in an industrial or business corporation. They are not the owners, nor do they have strong kinship ties with the owners. In the case of a hospital under the control and sponsorship of a religious order or a philanthropic group, they may not be members of the sponsoring group. They must make decisions with continual reference to their unwritten mandate: What do the owners or those in authority wish them to decide? The complexities of the decision-making process become evident when the participants and their distinct roles are identified and when the difficulties imposed by the mixed authority constellation in health care organizations are recognized.

EVALUATING A DECISION'S IMPORTANCE

By its nature, decision making means commitment. The importance of a decision may be measured in terms of the resources and time being committed. Some decisions affect only small segments of the organization, while others involve the entire organization. Some decisions are irrevocable because they create new situations. The degree of flexibility that remains after the commitment has been made may also be used in evaluating the signifi-cance of a decision: Are the resulting conditions tightly circumscribed, with little flexibility permitted, or are several options still available in developing subsequent plans? Decisions such as capital expenditures, major procedural systems, and the cost of the equipment that must be prorated over the pro-jected life of the equipment are examples.

The degree of certainty/uncertainty and, therefore, the degree of risk under which the decision is made is another dimension in weighing its im-pact. The greater the impact in terms of time, resources, and degree of risk, the more time, money, and effort must be directed toward making such decisions. Finally, in any organization, the impact on humans is a major factor. Environmental impact and social cost must be assessed.

STEPS IN DECISION MAKING

The decision-making process consists of several sequential steps: (1) agen-da building, including problem definition; (2) the search for alternatives; (3) evaluation of the alternatives; (4) commitment, i.e., the choice among alter-natives; and (5) continuing assessment of decisions, leading back to agenda building.

Agenda Building

Like planning, decision making may be viewed as a cyclic process. The first step, agenda building, flows from the feedback process. Information is gathered, clarified, and analyzed. The problem is defined and priorities as-signed. This step is critical, because subsequent decisions may be meaning-less and nonproductive unless the problem has been clarified. Indeed, the wrong problem may be solved, so to speak. Without problem clarification, a manager could implement a solution—possibly one that is costly in time, effort, and personnel—only to find recurring evidence and symptoms of the original problem, which remains unidentified and therefore unsolved.

For example, in a health center, there were long delays from the time of patient arrival until the time of treatment. The nursing and physician team felt under pressure because of patient complaints about the crowded waiting room and the long waits. The first effort to find a solution resulted in a triage system through which patients were assessed promptly and assigned priori-ties in the treatment process. In addition, considerable effort was made to improve the time allotments and sequencing of patients in the appointment system to help create a more orderly patient flow.

Having developed the triage system, changed the staffing pattern, and revamped the appointment system, the staff was faced with the same crowded waiting room. Why? During the second analysis, the true problem was identified. Because the transportation system in the local community was inadequate, patients tended to come to the center at the beginning of the day or at the end of the noon hour when family members were free to bring them. There was no other convenient way to get to the center. Furthermore, patients did not understand the appointment system process, nor did they believe that they would be seen at the appointed time.

When the health center, with the assistance of its community board, developed an alternate neighborhood transportation system, the problem was solved. Patient education programs concerning the appointment system were prepared, further helping to alleviate the problem.

Several management processes provide the executive with critical information for use in agenda building and problem identification. Analysis of the institution through use of the input-output model, for example, creates a systematic awareness of change in the organizational environment. Specific feedback processes, such as periodic formal reports and quality control routines, provide specific information for problem identification.

Search for Alternatives

Having defined and analyzed the problem, the decision maker searches for alternatives. It is the manager's job both to identify existing alternatives and to create new and better ones. The manager must remain open to all possible solutions to problems, taking care not to reject nontraditional approaches automatically. Alternatives may be identified quickly from past experience, but these must be accepted with caution because they may not fit the present situation. Creativity is a necessary element. An organizational climate of openness in which the development of original ideas is considered a legitimate use of the manager's time and effort fosters this approach. Coordinated time should be arranged for the management team as a whole, such as periodic team retreats during which day-to-day operations are set aside and the group assesses organizational needs and seeks creative approaches to satisfy these needs.

Chester Barnard, in his classic work on the functions of managers, stressed the importance of identifying the strategic or limiting factors that constrain the realistic development of alternatives.[3] The decision maker should confine the search for alternatives to those that will overcome these elements. This selectivity tends to prevent a waste of time and energy in developing alternatives that are infeasible and ineffective. Limiting factors that constrain decision making in health care include legal and accrediting standards, ethics, and lack of capital and trained personnel. The limiting or strategic factors change from time to time. Barnard saw the strategic factor as the point at which choice applies.[4] The solutions are narrowed to include only those that fit the organizational goals and availability of resources.

Evaluation of Alternatives

In order to evaluate alternatives, a manager must adopt an underlying philosophical stance, which includes a preliminary decision about the approach to decision making that will be taken. Depending on which philosophical stance is taken, certain alternatives will be acceptable and others excluded automatically. The philosophical approaches include the concepts of root and branch decisions, "satisficing" and maximizing, and the use of Paretian Optimality.

Root and Branch Decisions

Certain decisions are so fundamental to the organization's nature that their effects are pervasive and far-reaching in terms of organizational values, philosophy, goals, and overall policies. Such decisions, root decisions, invest the organization with its fundamental nature at its inception and carry it into periodic, comprehensive review of its fundamental purpose, often resulting in massive innovation. Thus, in the life cycle of an organization, root decisions may be associated with gestation when the fundamental form and purpose of the organization are crystallized. They may occur in middle age when new goals are developed and new organizational patterns are adopted. Finally, during old age and decline, a fundamental decision to dissolve the organization may be made. The pervasive effect of root decisions may be seen in the decision of a board of trustees to change a two-year college into a baccalaureate degree-granting institution or to convert a hospital into a multiple component health care center.

Charles Lindblom described root decisions and their opposite, branch or incremental decisions.[5] According to Lindblom, these incremental, limited, successive decisions do not involve a reevaluation of goals, policies, or underlying philosophy. Objectives and goals are recycled and policies are accepted without massive review and revision. Change is by degree. Only a small segment of the organization is affected.

Branch decision making is more conservative in its approach than is root decision making, with innovation inhibited. The stability of organizational life is enhanced, in many cases, when decision making is of the successive, incremental type, because the manager does not have the option of completely reviewing the organizational structure, functions, staffing patterns, equipment selection, and similar capital expenditures. Incrementalism also simplifies decision making because it tends to limit conflicts that might occur if the patterns of compromise, consensus, organizational territory, and subtle internal politics are disturbed. Incrementalism also may be the simple outcome of previous root decisions. On the other hand, the manager may overlook some excellent alternatives because they are not readily apparent in the chain of successive decisions. Incrementalism lacks the built-in safeguard of explicit, programmed review of values and philosophy.

Satisficing and Maximizing

"It might easily happen that what is second best is best, actually, because that which is actually best may be out of the question." This quotation, attributed to the philosopher-educator Cardinal Newman, expresses the idea contained in the concepts of satisficing and maximizing. In decision making, the one best solution may be determined by developing a set of criteria against which all alternatives are compared until one solution emerges as clearly preeminent. In maximizing as a part of decision making, this one best solution is the only acceptable one.

In satisficing, a term used by Simon,[6] a set of minimal criteria is developed, and any alternative that fulfills the minimal criteria is acceptable. A course of action that is good enough is selected, with the conscious recognition that there may be better solutions. When the manager seeks several options, satisficing may be employed. As with incrementalism, satisficing limits absolute, rational, optimal decision making, yet it simplifies the process. In satisficing, the manager accepts the fact that not every decision need be made with the same degree of intensity.

The Pareto Principle or Paretian Optimality

Vilfredo Pareto (1848–1923) was an Italian economist and sociologist who postulated a criterion for decision making that is referred to as the Pareto Principle or Paretian Optimality.[7] He suggested that each person's needs be met as much as possible without any loss to another person. In this mode of decision making, certain alternatives are rejected because of the decrease in benefits for one or several groups. Decisions that result in a major gain for one individual with concomitant major loss for another are avoided. The approach involves compromise and consensus, with each manager accepting the needs of other units of the organization as legitimate and the needs of the organization as a whole as paramount. The concessions and trade-offs in the budget process or in the labor negotiation process illustrate the balance required to satisfy the needs of many departments or groups without penalizing any one or at least penalizing all departments or groups in equal measure.

Commitment Phase

In the definition of decision making, the essential focus is choice—the specific selection from among alternatives. At some point, deliberation must be ended. If a manager does not make a decision in a timely way, someone else may make the decision. In some rare cases, managers find that alternatives are of equal merit. Should that occur, the manager can simply follow personal preference.

The commitment phase can be divided into stages: the pilot run and sequential implementation. A pilot run to test the chosen alternative helps reduce the risk attached to the decision. For example, a manufacturing company may offer a new product on trial and make further decisions based on the results. Rather than purchasing expensive equipment, managers may choose a leasing arrangement with an option to purchase. Pilot runs have two distinct limitations, however; they are costly in terms of time and money, and they are not always feasible.

In sequential implementation, managers make a basic determination and assess the result before they take the next step in the implementation process. The cycle is shortened; feedback is obtained and alternatives reviewed and implemented after a relatively short time. During the implementation stage, the decisions must be communicated to those who will carry out the detailed plans that flow from it.

Continuing Assessment of Decisions

The final step in the decision-making process is the continuous analysis of the decision. Through the feedback process, a new agenda is generated and new alternatives revealed. The steps in the control process provide a link back to the planning and decision-making functions.

BARRIERS TO RATIONAL CHOICE

Managers must recognize that there are barriers to rational choice and that it may not be possible to make the perfect decision because of these subtle barriers. One set of barriers stems from human nature itself—ignorance, prejudice, and resistance to change all influence decision making. If managers do not have the necessary information or if they have it but cannot make use of it because they lack proper training in analytical skills, their ability to make informed decisions is circumscribed. Prejudice, i.e., preconceived opinion, is another aspect of human nature that must be taken into account. Even with sufficient factual knowledge, the value elements in decisions are inescapable. Resistance to change constitutes a third such barrier; managers may continue to make decisions based on their own past experience.

Together, these barriers constitute an overall impediment: inadequate leadership. Leaders may fail to take risks, choosing the security of incremental change. They may stifle creative thinking in themselves and their subordinates. They may so limit their zone of acceptance that change becomes difficult and decisions by precedent become the only decisions possible. They may ignore feedback, thus reinforcing their own positions and making determinations based on limited facts that are colored by their own value premises.

The internal dynamics of the decision-making process have been studied by psychologists Irving L. Janis and Leon Mann.[8] They identified four situations in which the decision maker fails to reach the ideal of "vigilant information processing":

1. If the risks involved in continuing to do whatever has been done in the past appear low, the individual is likely to go on doing it and is unlikely to collect adequate information about possible alternatives.
2. If the risks of continuing to do whatever has been done in the past appear high and if the risks of an obvious alternative appear low, the decision maker is likely to choose the obvious alternative and again is unlikely to collect adequate information about other possibilities.
3. If all the obvious alternatives seem to involve risk and if the decision maker feels that there is little chance of coming up with a better alternative, the individual is likely to engage in "defensive avoidance" by denying that a problem exists, to exaggerate the advantage of the chosen alternative, or to try to get someone else to make the decision.
4. If the decision maker feels that there is a potentially satisfactory course of action and that this alternative may disappear if there is a delay to investigate other possibilities, the individual is likely to panic, trying to pursue the obvious alternative before it is too late.

Decision makers undertake "vigilant information processing" only if they feel that all the obvious choices are risky, that there may be a better choice that is not obvious, and that there is sufficient time to seek the best possible choice.

Other barriers to rational choice flow from the organizational structure. There may be so much organizational red tape that decision making is limited to decision by precedent. Department managers may lack sufficient authority to make decisions and may be required to submit to a committee process for some decisions. Decisions made in other departments may, in turn, affect their own, but they may have no influence in those areas. There may be a lack of sufficient coordination in decision making throughout the organization. Organizational politics, e.g., bargaining, forming alliances, and choosing "the right time," also subtly limits rational decision making.

Factors related to the social, political, and economic climate outside the organization also act as barriers. The many aspects of law and regulation governing health care set specific limits, for example. Finally, the degree of certainty under which decisions are made tends to impose limits on choice. Under conditions of high certainty, the risk involved in decision making is low, and decisions may become routine. After they have been standardized through the use of policy, procedures, and rules, routine decisions may be made at lower levels of the organization. Conditions of relative certainty/uncertainty obviously increase risk, and managers attempt to evaluate alternatives in terms of probable payoff. The decision maker's efforts focus on reducing the risk and on developing, as far as possible, quantifiers with which to measure the probable payoff. Statistical analysis of data, market research, and forecasting are a few of the decision-making tools that may be employed in assessing comparative probability. Decisions made under great uncertainty involve the highest level of risk, and the burden for making such decisions belongs to the top echelons of the organization.

BASES FOR DECISION MAKING

Since effective decision making is critical to organizational survival, managers seek to overcome the barriers to rational choice. The bases for decision making range from intuition and serendipity to research and analysis. The manager's previous experience may be a valid basis for decisions, provided that there are no changes in the constraints nor in the goals to be reached. Managers may draw from the experiences of other, similar organizations. This "copy your neighbor" or "follow the leader" approach may provide managers with information they do not have available. For example, another organization may have research information available, or a manager in another institution may have explored alternatives in great detail so that others could profit from such an analysis. A manager may take the philosophical attitude that it is not necessary to reinvent the wheel and that it is wise to learn from others; however, not only are these approaches based on an assumption that the managers being copied are correct in their decisions, but also they do not take into account the different constraints under which each manager operates.

The creative approach to decision making seeks to capitalize on intuition and serendipity, but they must be augmented by more concrete analysis of information before final determinations are made. Experimentation, research, and analysis constitute the most effective base for selecting among alternatives.

DECISION-MAKING TOOLS AND TECHNIQUES

Managers have available the historical records, information about past performance, and summaries of their own and other managers' experience. In addition, managers may test alternatives through the use of decision-making tools and techniques.

Considered Opinion and Devil's Advocate

A manager may obtain the considered opinion of experts and use the technique of "the devil's advocate" to sharpen the arguments for and against an alternative. In the first instance, the manager asks staff experts or other members of the management team to assess the several alternatives and develop arguments for and against each; the resulting comparative assessment helps the decision maker to select a course of action.

When the devil's advocate technique is used, the decision maker assigns an individual or group the duty of developing statements of all the negative aspects or weaknesses of each alternative. Each potential decision is tested through frank discussion of weaknesses and error before the proposed action is implemented. The underlying theory is that it is better to subject decisions to strict, internal, organized criticism than to run the risk of having a hidden weakness or error exposed after a decision has been implemented. The devil's advocate does not make a judgment, but simply develops arguments to ensure that all aspects are considered.

The Factor Analysis Matrix

For the decision maker who must overcome personal preference to make an impartial decision, the matrix of comparative factors is an effective tool of analysis. As a first step, the decision maker develops the criteria under two major categories: essential elements (musts) and desired elements (wants).

The choices available are compared through the development of a table or matrix. The factors can be assigned relative weight, as in a point scale, and the alternative with the highest point value becomes the best option. Even without the weighting factors, the matrix remains useful as a technique of factual comparison. Table 4–1 illustrates the use of the must and want categories to compare equipment for departmental use. A similar process could be used to evaluate applicants for a job; personal bias can be set aside more easily and candidates compared on the basis of their qualifications for the position (Table 4–2).

The Decision Tree

A managerial tool used to depict the possible directions that actions might take from various decision points, the decision tree forces the manager to ask the "what then" questions, i.e., to anticipate outcomes. Possible events are included, with a notation about the probabilities associated with each. The basic decisions are stated, with all the unfolding, probable events branching out from them. The decision tree enables managers to undertake disciplined speculation about the consequences, including the unpleasant or negative ones, of actions. Through the use of the decision tree, managers are forced to delineate their reasoning, and the constraints imposed by probable future events on subsequent decisions become evident. The decision tree reveals the probable new situation that results from a decision.

Table 4–1 Matrix of Comparison for Equipment Purchase

	Brand A	Brand B	Brand C
* Maximum cost	Acceptable	Acceptable	$100+
* Compatibility with related equipment	Yes	Yes	No
* Minimum years of service	No	Yes	Yes
* Availability of service	Yes	Yes	Yes
* Renovation of existing space not needed	Yes	Needed	Yes
O Safety features	Yes	Yes	Yes
O Trade-in value for present equipment	No	No	Yes
O Available delivery date	Yes	No	Yes
O Special training for use	No	Yes	Yes
O Lease option	No	No	Yes

* = must;   O = want.

Table 4-2 Matrix for Evaluation of Job Applicants

	Applicant A	Applicant B	Applicant C
* Type at 60 wpm	40 wpm	50	60
* Transcription of medical reports at 800 lines/day	600	600	750
Previous experience this type job	0	1 yr.	1 yr.
Knowledge of related clerical job	Telephone unit clerk	same	
Organizational policy: preference for internal applicants	3 yrs.	1 yr.	0
* Willing to accept salary of $12,010	yes	yes	Prefers higher; wants raise within six months
* Full time	yes	yes	
* 3 P.M. to 10 P.M. shift acceptable	yes	yes	Prefers day; plans to switch as soon as opening is available

* Must/essential

It is possible to use the decision tree without including mathematical calculations of probability, although computers are commonly used to calculate the probability of events when such detailed information is available. Managers in business corporations with sufficient market data about profit, loss, patterns of consumer response, and national economic fluctuations include these data in the construction of a decision tree for the marketing of a new product, for example.

Managers who lack detailed information of this type can still use the decision tree to advantage. In developing a decision tree, these managers use symbols to designate points of certainty and uncertainty. For example, events of certainty may be placed in rectangles; events of uncertainty, in ovals. This technique emphasizes the relative risk in each decision track. The goal to be reached is the continual reference point. The sequence of decisions that leads to the goal with the least uncertainty emerges as a distinct track, thereby facilitating the manager's decision. For decisions in which the manager has intense personal involvement, this approach is a valuable aid in overcoming emotional barriers to objective choice.

Operations Research

During World War II, operations research was developed when the military in Britain and in the United States faced massive logistical problems. Because there was not enough time to carry out research and trial runs, conditions were simulated in models that permitted greater experimentation. Management literature contains three terms, used interchangeably at times, that reflect this process of model building to analyze decision alternatives: *operational research, operations research,* and *management science.* Operational research, the earliest term used, was shortened to operations research as the processes were applied to business practices. Operations research is also referred to under the broad term of management science.

The use of operations research, with its extensive mathematical analyses and probability calculations, became broadly feasible with the development of computer technology. By definition, operations research is an applied science in which the scientific method is brought to bear on a problem, process, or operation. It is a technique for quantitative problem solving and decision making in which mathematical models are applied to management problems. Three major steps are included in operations research techniques:

1. problem formulation. The problem is stated and preconceived notions are set aside.

2. construction of a mathematical or conceptual model. This is usually done through equations or formulas representing and relating critical factors in the problem under analysis.
3. manipulation of variables. This is done to develop and assess alternatives in terms of designated criteria.

Simulation and Model Building

Simulation is the representation of a process or system by means of a model. A model is a logical, simplified representation of an aspect of reality. Models range from simple, as in a physical form, to complex, as in mathematical equations. Since legal, ethical, and economic constraints limit the manipulation of reality, experimentation may be carried out on the representation of reality, i.e., the model, rather than on reality itself. Through the development of models, managers attempt to gain additional information about the uncertainties in the situation; those elements are brought into focus and assessments made concerning the degree of chance associated with them.

Managers use several models routinely. For example, they may use a physical model of the office layout, reducing in scale the dimensions of the office space and equipment. During an in-service training session, a manager in a health-related profession may use one or several physical models, such as a model of a body organ. An organization chart is a graphic model of departmental and authority relationships. A decision tree is a schematic model of plans or decisions. Analog and mathematical models are the most complex, with mathematical models the most abstract. Some models are developed through reasoning by analogy (analog model); a problem is approached indirectly by setting up an analogous situation, solving it, and making a similar application to the original problem. The model for one problem is converted into a form suitable for a different problem.

Stochastic Simulation

A model designed to include the element of randomness is called a stochastic simulation model. Stochastic is derived from the Greek word meaning guess or not certain. The Monte Carlo method is a form of stochastic simulation in which data are developed through the random number generator. Where the variables are uncertain, at least a sample of their values may be assigned through the development of a statistical pattern of distribution. In this way, managers may simulate such occurrences as employee absenteeism, patient arrivals, or equipment failures. The Monte Carlo technique involves factors of change and their effect on the process or system. Probability sampling is used extensively with simulation and model building.

Waiting Line and Queuing Theory

In any organization in which the demand for service fluctuates, managers must balance the cost of waiting lines with the cost of preventing waiting lines through increased service. Waiting lines or queues are a common, everyday experience: customers in a grocery store, cars at a toll gate, airplanes stacked to land, patients in a clinic or emergency room, telephone requests for information. A characteristic of such queues is the randomness of demand. Waiting line or queuing theory is useful for analyzing those situations in which the units to be provided for the service are relatively predictable. The underlying premise is that delays are costly; yet, too little activity on another occasion is also costly. For example, hospital emergency room resources are costly when not used; however, the cost in terms of patient pain, aggravation, and inconvenience must be taken into account if an emergency arises and there is a delay in treatment.

There are three basic components in waiting line analysis: arrivals, servicing, and queue discipline. The unit of arrival is defined, e.g., grocery orders to be rung up, planes to be landed, patients to be examined. The pattern of arrival is studied to determine probabilities of arrival. Arrivals can be divided into three categories:

1. predetermined arrivals, such as scheduled airplane landings or scheduled patient appointments
2. random arrivals, such as emergency landings at an airport or patient arrivals at a walk-in clinic or emergency unit
3. combination of predetermined and random arrivals, such as arrivals at a clinic with both scheduled appointments and a walk-in system

Servicing is the focus of analysis of the workflow; the service is defined in terms of number of units and time needed for each pattern of distribution. Analysis of these data shows both random and constant factors that must be taken into account when procedures are developed. Various control processes are developed to smooth these internal activities. Queue discipline involves an analysis of the patterns or characteristics of the waiting line, such as average minimum and maximum wait, the number of lines, the manner in which units are selected for service (e.g., first come, first served; random selection; triage system according to severity of problem or ease of processing; priority and preference system). Through the analysis of such information, managers can make informed decisions to overcome the negative aspects of waiting lines (delay for patients) and the cost to the organization (idle equipment, overstaffing).

Gaming and Game Theory

Gaming is the simulation of competitive situations in which the element of uncertainty is introduced as a result of some other, often competing, decision maker's action. In the management field, games give reality to training situations and to the decision-making process. Unlike other forms of simulation, gaming uses human decisions, although they may be computer-assisted.

Game theory is a branch of mathematical analysis of conflict and strategy; it is associated with the concepts of zero sum games and minimax strategy. Both involve theoretical situations in which competitive conditions are central; they are based on the premises that each competitor acts rationally and seeks to maximize gain, to minimize loss, and to outwit the other competitors. Game theory remains relatively undeveloped because of the complexities that arise once the number of contestants or rules is increased.

Gaming and game theory are separate, distinct concepts, although somewhat related. These techniques of operations research are costly means of testing alternatives, yet they are less expensive than a monumental mistake. By making dry runs possible, these methods clarify the size of the risks.

THE HEALTH CARE PRACTITIONER AS DECISION MAKER

The professional health care practitioner in the managerial role faces decision-making situations on a routine basis. Decision making takes place within the dynamics of organizational structure, and strategy is an essential part of the process. Not all decisions are presented to managers in clear-cut fashion. The elements of decision making are embodied in the following cases drawn from typical management situations in a health care setting.

> Helen R. is an experienced home health administrator. An O.T.R. with a master's degree in business administration and 15 years of experience, she recently joined the staff of a nonprofit home health agency as its Director of Professional Services. Her duties include the supervision of nurses, physical therapists, occupational therapists, and home health aides. She realized that several hurdles would have to be overcome if the full authority of the position were to be realized. For example, Helen observed that she

would have to change the informal power structure of the agency if she wanted to fulfill her formal role.

The factors that Helen found were these:

1. The management of the agency consisted of the owner/director and his wife. Both had experience in operating a wholesale grocery store, but neither had any experience in health care delivery.
2. Madeline B. managed the nursing and home health aide units. She was efficient and knowledgeable, but she seemed controlling and tactless during supervisory meetings. Staff rarely remained with the agency for more than 11 months.
3. Madeline avoided Helen and never talked about patient care matters.
4. The agency contracted for physical therapy services from a private practice group. These practitioners were not employees of the agency.
5. Occupational therapy services also were obtained from private practice groups on a contract basis.

Helen confirmed her observations during the next two weeks. She listed her priorities: (1) to increase her visibility in the social system by establishing her credibility as an expert and (2) to fashion an appropriate role for the Director of Professional Services.

Initially, Helen did not have the power to assume the duties of her role formally. The director and his wife not only seemed uninterested in helping her, but also appeared not to understand why they had hired her, other than a general recognition that the agency "ought to have a director of professional services because several other agencies had such a position." Since Madeline enjoyed so much informal power, Helen would have to build her own role over a period of time.

To solidify her formal position, Helen developed a strategy. She would offer her expert opinions to the director and his wife. These would be cost-effective and at the same time benefit her own position. Helen decided to avoid direct confrontation with Madeline until she had accrued more status in the organization. Helen's ability to select her issues marks her as an experienced manager. The decision to increase her status as she created more income for the agency was a creative use of opportunity and resources.

Helen accomplished her goal by role expansion. She hired three occupational therapists and two speech pathologists. She selected her contract professionals carefully, hiring individuals who would support her in her role as Director of Professional Services. The introduction of new services increased the agency's revenues. Because of the increase in patient referrals, Helen added a second nursing supervisor, making sure that this nursing supervisor also accepted Helen's role as overall Director of Professional Services. Madeline's informal power was thus diluted by a series of formal and informal actions. Helen's decisions were calculated risks.

A second example offered here for analysis is presented in a summary form to highlight the decision-making elements:

1. Problem Definition.
   a. Whether to retain John J., staff therapist, or lay him off.
   b. Background of the problem:
      1. John is the senior therapist in the rehabilitation department of a municipal hospital. He has worked at the hospital for seven years.
      2. John's work has been deteriorating over the past two years. He comes to work late, is slow to start, takes numerous breaks, and does not seem interested in his patients.
      3. John has been absent from work without telephoning to report the reason. This has created bad feelings among the other staff, as it makes last minute scheduling changes necessary.
      4. John's supervisor has discussed his situation with him every other week for the past six months. She would like to offer him an extended leave at half pay until he is "better."
2. Search for Alternatives. The supervisor made an appointment with the physician-director of rehabilitation services. Together, they searched for alternatives:
   a. Give employee formal notice of unsatisfactory performance, stipulating that, if he fails to improve, he will be placed on probation.
   b. Offer (and insist) that employee enter a counseling program offered to employees.
   c. Demote employee with subsequent decrease in pay and benefits.
   d. Leave employee alone to work out his problems.

3. Evaluation of Alternatives.
   a. Giving him notice seems drastic since he has senior status. This alternative could be used later, if other measures fail.
   b. Counseling seems most promising, but what happens if employee refuses to enter the program?
   c. Demotion requires much documentation and does not address the real problem.
   d. Leaving employee alone has been tried, and the results were not successful.
4. Commitment: Choice of Alternatives.
   a. Offer employee the option of seeking counseling. Stipulation is made that his work must improve or he must suffer the consequences. Employee was given a written summary of this conference.
   b. Other alternatives are eliminated at present time.
5. Assessment.
   a. Employee's performance is monitored and appropriate documentation developed over specified time frame.
   b. If employee's performance does not improve, supervisor must begin the decision-making cycle again, redefining the problem and assessing alternatives in the light of new information.

NOTES

1. Herbert Simon, *Administrative Behavior* (New York: MacMillan, 1957), Preface and Chapter 1.

2. Ibid.

3. Chester Barnard, *The Functions of the Executive* (Cambridge, MA: Harvard University Press, 1968), p. 202.

4. Ibid., p. 205.

5. Charles Lindblom, "The Science of Muddling Through," *Public Administration Review,* Spring, 1959, pp. 79–88.

6. Herbert Simon, *Models of Man* (New York: John Wiley & Sons, 1957), p. 207.

7. Vilfredo Pareto, *Mind and Society* (New York: Harcourt, Brace, and Co., 1935).

8. Irving L. Janis and Leon Mann, *A Psychological Analysis of Conflict, Choice and Commitment* (New York: The Free Press, 1978).

Chapter 5

Organizing

CHAPTER OBJECTIVES

1. Define the management function of organizing.
2. Identify the basic steps in the process of organizing.
3. Define key concepts: hierarchy, chain of command, splintered authority, concurring authority.
4. Cite factors that shape the span of management.
5. Differentiate between line and staff relationships.
6. Identify basic line and staff relationships.
7. Recognize the dual pyramid arrangement in health care patterns of authority.
8. Identify the basic patterns of departmentation.
9. Relate temporary departmentation and matrix organization to the need for organizational flexibility.
10. Identify the principles for constructing an organization chart.
11. Identify the elements of job description development.
12. Identify the uses of the job description.

Organizing is the process of grouping the necessary responsibilities and activities into workable units, determining the lines of authority and communication, and developing patterns of coordination. It is the conscious development of role structures of superior and subordinate, line and staff. The organizational process stems from the following underlying premises:

• There is a common goal toward which work effort is directed.

• The goal is spelled out in detailed plans.

• There is need for clear authority-responsibility relationships.

- Power and authority elements must be reconciled so that individual interactions within the organization are productive and goal-directed.

- Conflict is inevitable but may be reduced through clarity of organizational relationships.

- Individual needs must be reconciled with and subordinated to the organizational needs.

- Unity of command must prevail.

- Authority must be delegated.

THE PROCESS OF ORGANIZING

The immediately identifiable aspects of the organizational process include clear delineation of the goal in terms of scope, function, and priorities. For example, will a health care institution focus on acute care for inpatients or comprehensive care, including outpatient care, even home care? Will the organization expand its services through decentralized locations and active outreach programs?

The development of specific organizational structure must be considered. What degree of specialization will be sought? Specialization is a major feature of health care organizations; it is dictated and shaped in part by the specific licensure mandates for each health profession. The manager must assess the question of line and staff officers and units. A major organizational question concerns the division of work. What will be the pattern of departmentation? The development of the organization chart, the job descriptions, and the statements of interdepartmental and intradepartmental workflow systems must be assessed and implemented as part of the management function of organizing. Finally, the changes in the internal and external organization environment must be monitored so that the organizational structure can be adjusted accordingly.

In summary, the basic steps of organizing are

1. goal recognition and statement
2. review of organizational environment
3. determination of structure needed to reach the goal (e.g., degree of centralization, basis of departmentation, committee use, line and staff relationships)
4. determination of authority relationships and development of the organization chart, job descriptions, and related support documents

FUNDAMENTAL CONCEPTS AND PRINCIPLES

Relationships in formal organizations are highly structured in terms of authority and responsibility. The resulting hierarchy, i.e., the arrangement of individuals into a graded series of superiors and subordinates, authority holders, and rank and file members, constitutes one of the most obvious characteristics of formal organizations. A pyramid-shaped organization tends to result from the development of hierarchy (Figure 5–1).

The flow of authority and responsibility that can be observed in the hierarchy constitutes a distinct chain of command, also referred to as the scalar principle: the chain of direct authority from superior to subordinate. Unity of command can be expected to prevail. Unity of command is the uninterrupted line of authority from superior to subordinate so that each individual reports to one, and only one, superior. A clear chain of command shows who reports to whom, who is responsible for the actions of an individual, who has authority over the worker.

The authority delegated to any individual must be equal to the responsibility assigned. This principle of parity—that responsibility cannot be greater

Figure 5–1 Pyramidal Hierarchy

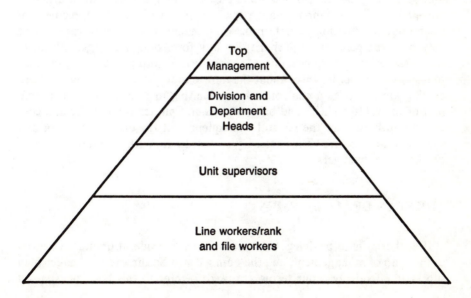

Top Management

Division and Department Heads

Unit supervisors

Line workers/rank and file workers

than the authority given—ensures that individuals can carry out their assigned duties without provoking conflict over their right to do so. In developing policies and documents that support the organization chart, managers must avoid contradicting this principle of parity. At the same time, managers cannot so completely delegate authority that they become free of responsibility. This is reflected in the principle of the absoluteness of responsibility; authority may (and must) be delegated, but ultimate responsibility is retained by the manager. This, in turn, is the basis of the manager's right to exercise the necessary controls and require accountability.

Normally, managers have adequate authority to carry out the required activities of their divisions or units without recourse to the authority mandate of other managers. Two situations occur, however, in which the authority of a single manager is not sufficient for unilateral decision making or action. Occasionally, because the work must be coordinated and because there are necessary limits on each manager's authority, a problem cannot be solved or a decision made without pooling the authority of two or more managers. These problems of splintered authority are overcome in three ways: (1) the managers may simply pool their authority and make the decision or solve the problem; (2) the problem may be referred to a higher level of authority until it reaches one manager with sufficient authority; or (3) reorganization may be done so that recurring situations of splintered authority are eliminated. Such recurring situations sometimes require adjustment in the permanent authority delegation.

Concurring authority is sometimes given to related departments to ensure uniformity of practice. For example, the packaging department of a manufacturing company cannot change specifications without the agreement of the production division. A data processing manager in a health care setting may be given concurring authority on any form design changes, although this is the primary responsibility of the medical record practitioner, in order to foster compatibility throughout the information processing function. Concurring authority, as a control and coordinating measure, can be a normal part of the routine check and balance system. Splintered authority and concurring authority are the natural consequences of the division of labor and specialization that make it necessary to coordinate authority delegations of two or more managers.

THE SPAN OF MANAGEMENT

If authority is to be delegated appropriately, consideration must be given to the span of management, i.e., the number of subordinates a manager may supervise effectively. Four terms are used to refer to this concept: *span of*

management, span of control, span of supervision, and *span of authority.*
Stated another way, the span of management is the number of immediate
subordinates who report to any one manager. It is essential to recognize that
the number of individuals whose activities can be properly coordinated and
controlled by one manager is limited.

There is no ideal span of management, although the numbers of 4 or 5
persons at higher levels and 8 or 12 at the lower levels have been suggested.
Modifying factors shape the appropriate span of management for any authority holder, however. These factors include

- the type of work. Routine, repetitive, homogeneous work allows a larger
  span of management.

- the degree of training of the worker. Those who are well trained and well
  motivated do not need as much supervision as a trainee group; the more
  highly trained the group, the larger the span of management may be.

- organizational stability. When the organization as a whole, as well as the
  specific department, is stable, the span of control can be wider; when
  there are rapid changes, high turnover, and general organizational insta-
  bility, a more narrow span of control may be needed.

- geographical location. When the work units are dispersed over a scat-
  tered physical layout, sometimes even involving separate geographical
  locations, closer supervision is necessary to control and coordinate the
  work.

- flow of work. If much coordination of work flow is needed, there is a
  companion need for greater supervision, a narrow span of control.

- supervisor's qualifications. As the degree of training and amount of experience of the supervisor increase, the span of control for that supervisor
  may increase also.

- availability of staff specialists. When staff specialists and selected support services, such as a training or personnel development department,
  are available, a supervisor's span of management may be widened.

- the value system of the organization. In highly coercive organizations, a
  supervisor may have a large span of management, since there is a pervasive system to help ensure conformity, even to the extent of severe punishment for deviation from the rules. In a highly normative organization,
  however, there may be an emphasis on participation in planning and
  decision making and a resultant complexity in the communication process; thus, a smaller span of management may be appropriate. In health
  care organizations, a traditionally normative setting with respect to the
  professional worker, the span of management may be large because the

health care professional is a specialist within an area and does not always require close supervision.

As an example, the span of management in an occupational therapy department is shown in Figure 5–2. The relationship of other units in the division, as well as the relationship of the division to other divisions in the organization, can be seen.

Figure 5–2 Organizational Chart of Bentwood Hospital for Children

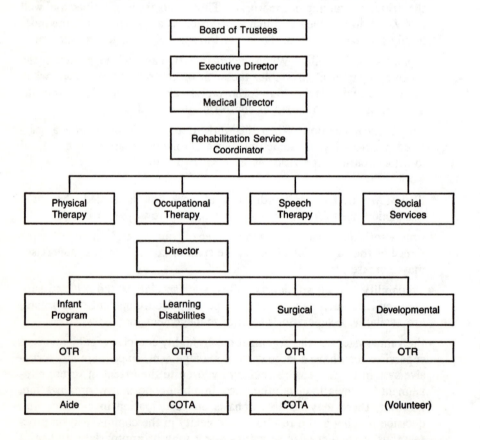

Note: OTR, Occupational Therapist Registered; COTA, Certified Occupational Therapy Assistant.

LINE AND STAFF RELATIONSHIPS

The terms *line* and *staff* are key words in any discussion of organizing. In common usage, staff refers to the groups of employees who perform the work of a given department or unit. The director of nurses speaks of the nursing staff, the chief dietitian discusses the dietary staff, and the physicians who practice in a hospital are referred to as the medical staff.

In management literature, a differentiation is made between line and staff departments or officers. Line refers only to those that have direct responsibility for accomplishing the objectives of the organization; staff, to those that help the line units achieve the objectives. In a health care organization, direct patient care units are considered the line functions, and all other units are listed as staff services. The problem with this distinction becomes apparent when it must be applied to such units as the dietary, purchasing, or housekeeping departments; are these functions any less essential to the operation of a health care organization than a direct patient care unit? Some authors prefer to list such units as service departments, reserving staff for a specific authority relationship.

The concept of line and staff was inherited by management theorists from the military of the 18th and 19th centuries. An examination of a military encounter typical in these eras makes it easier to conceptualize these aspects of line and staff. The soldiers literally formed a line; the immediate commanding officers were those who commanded the line, that is, line officers. The actual fighting of the battle was the duty of these troops and officers. In turn, these troops and officers were assisted by staff officers and other units that provided logistical support, supplies, and information. The idea carried over as formal bureaucratic organizational theory developed in the 19th century.

Line and Staff as Authority Relationship

The term *staff* also involves statements of relationships in the authority domain. Again, the original usage of the term was derived from the military, in which the staff assistant pattern was developed as a means of relieving commanders of details that could be handled by others. The staff officer was an "assistant to" the commander, and this assistant was an extension of line authority. Such a relationship tends to be manager to manager.

The essence of line authority is a direct chain of command or line from the top level of authority through each successive level of the organization. A manager with line authority has direct authority and responsibility for the work of a unit; the line manager alone has the right to command others to act. A staff assistant provides advice, counsel, or technical support that may be accepted, altered, or rejected by the line officer.

Functional authority is the right of individuals to exercise a limited form of authority over the specialized functions for which they are responsible, regardless of who exercises line authority over the employees performing the activities. For example, the data processing staff is responsible for developing and implementing a specific computerized data collection system. The unit manager has functional authority over processing input documents, although these documents may be originated and completed by workers in other units, such as the admission office, business office, nursing service, or medical record service. A personnel officer may be charged with monitoring organizational compliance with affirmative action programs or labor union contracts; the advice of such an officer could not be rejected or altered arbitrarily by a line officer.

A staff officer or manager may hold a staff position. Such an individual may be the designated officer in charge of a support department, such as legal counsel or personnel. Yet, this manager may also have charge of one or several workers within the unit and would exercise line authority within that unit. Organization charts, job descriptions, and similar documents should contain clear statements as to the nature of each position: line or staff, kind of authority, and area of responsibility.

Line and Staff Interaction

Various types of staff arrangements may be developed to channel line and staff interaction. As noted earlier, one basic mode of interaction is to designate a staff member as the personal assistant to an individual holding office in the upper levels of the organization. This position should not be confused with that of an assistant department head or assistant manager, who generally shares in direct line authority. Managers in the upper levels of the organization may have several assistants, each carrying out highly specialized tasks. When there is only one position of assistant, this individual's work may be general, varied, and determined by the needs of the superior officer. The style of interaction may be highly personal, as when the staff assistant is seen as an alter ego of the line officer. When such a staff member indicates a point of view, a desired action, or a preferred decision, other members of the organization recognize that this individual is reflecting the opinion and wishes of the line officer.

A full department that gives specialized assistance and support frequently has a general staff. The relationship between staff and line personnel is less intimate than the assistant relationship. The work tends to be technical and highly specialized, as in the military's use of a logistical staff.

A third aspect of line and staff relationship is the organizational arrangement of the specialized staff: this individual (or department in a large institution) gives highly specialized counsel, such as that provided by an engineer, architect, accountant, lawyer, or auditor. Finally, as noted, departments can be arranged in terms of direct line entities, assisted by support or service units.

DUAL PYRAMID OF ORGANIZATION IN HEALTH CARE

Health care institutions are characterized by a dual pyramid of organization because of the traditional relationship of the medical staff to the administrative staff. The ultimate authority and responsibility for the management of the institution is vested in the governing board. In accordance with the stipulations of licensure and accrediting agencies, the board appoints a chief executive officer (administrator) and a chief of medical staff, resulting in two lines of authority. The chief executive officer is responsible for effectively managing the administrative components of the institution and delegates authority to each department head in the administrative component. Within the administrative units, there is a typical pyramidal organization with a unified chain of command.

The physicians and dentists are organized under a specific set of bylaws for the governance of the medical and dental staff. With governing board approval, the chief of the medical staff appoints the chief of each clinical service. Physicians and dentists apply for clinical privileges through the medical staff credentials committee and receive appointment from the governing board. A second pyramid results from this organization of the medical staff into clinical services, with each having a chief of service who reports to the chief of the medical staff.

In an effort to consolidate authority and clarify responsibility, the top administrative levels of a health care organization may be expanded to include a central officer to whom both the administrator and the chief of the medical staff report. In some institutions, however, there may be no permanent medical staff position that corresponds to the position of administrator on the organization chart. The elected president of the medical staff may fill this role when there is no organizational slot for a medical director per se. It is important to determine the precise meaning of titles as they are used in a specific health care setting. The following are titles commonly used:

• chief of staff: an officer of the medical staff to whom the chiefs of medical and clinical services report; appointed by the governing board.

- chief of service: physician-director of specific clinical service, e.g., chief of surgery; the line officer for physicians who are appointed to the specific service.
- chairman of department: physician-director of specific clinical service in an academic institution, such as a teaching hospital. (This title may be used as an alternate to chief of service in this type of setting.)
- medical director: full-time position in line authority structure; sometimes seen as the counterpart of the chief executive officer for the medical staff.
- president of the medical staff: presiding officer for the medical staff, usually elected for a year. In the absence of a full-time medical director, this individual serves as coordinating officer for the medical staff.

Although all authority flows from the governing board, there are two distinct chains of command, one in the administrative structure and one in the medical/clinical sector. Furthermore, in matters of direct patient care, the attending physician exercises professional authority; thus, a single employee not only may be subject to more than one line of authority, but also may have professional authority. Line officers in the administrative unit may find that their authority is limited in some areas because of the specific jurisdiction of the medical staff committees, such as the pharmacy and therapeutics committee. The director of the physical therapy department, for example, may report to a committee of physicians of the active medical staff, which limits the authority mandate of this line manager. Because of the dual pyramid structure, much coordination is needed.

BASIC DEPARTMENTATION

The development of departments is a natural adjunct to the division of labor and specialization that are characteristics of formal organizations. Departmentation overcomes the limitation imposed by the span of management. The organization, through its departments and similar subdivisions, can expand almost indefinitely in size. Departmentation facilitates the coordination process, since there is a logical grouping of closely related activities. Basic departmentation may be developed according to any one of several patterns:

1. by function. Because it is logical, efficient, and natural, the most widely used form of departmentation is to group all the related activities or jobs together. This permits managers to take advantage of specialization and to concern themselves with only one major focus of activity. Hospital departments are usually developed according to the pattern of

functional departmentation, e.g., business office and medical records, personnel, housekeeping, maintenance, and dietary departments.

2. by product. All activities needed in the development, production, and marketing of a product may be grouped for coordination and control. This pattern of departmentation is used in business and industry where one or a few closely related products are grouped. It facilitates the use of research funds, specialized skills and knowledge, and the development of cost control data for each product line. Functional departmentation may be an adjunct of product departmentation.

3. by territory. In business, the marketing process may be developed according to geographical boundaries. In service organizations, a decentralized pattern based on customer/client groupings may be appropriate. In some health care organizations, territorial departmentation is used because funding stipulations designate specific catchment areas or require coverage of certain population centers. Local needs, such as participation of clients and prompt settlement of difficulties, may be accommodated more easily through departmentation by territory. Grouping by geographical territory is a common element in outreach programs and home care services, as it fosters efficient movement of personnel to client location.

4. by customer. Departmentation may be based on client need. Specialty clinics in health care tend to follow this pattern. Government programs frequently focus on specific client need, partly in response to the lobbying of interest groups. Specific examples of customer/client departmentation include special maternal and infant care programs, the Veterans Administration, and programs for migrant workers. A university may have components such as day, evening, and weekend divisions, as well as continuing education programs, to accommodate the needs and interests of differing student populations.

5. by time. Activities may be grouped according to the time of day they are performed. Usually referred to as the use of shifts within the normal workday, this pattern is common in manufacturing and similar organizations in which the activities of a relatively large group of semi-skilled or technical workers are repetitive and continue around the clock. Organizations that provide essential services throughout the day and night use this pattern, usually in conjunction with functional departmentation.

6. by process. Technological considerations and specialized equipment usage may lead to departmentation by process. It is similar to functional departmentation in that all the activities involving one major process or some specialized equipment are grouped. In health care organizations,

the formation of radiology or clinical laboratory departments illustrates a form of departmentation by process as well as by function.

7. by number. Departmentation may be done by assigning certain duties to undifferentiated workers under specific supervision. This form of departmentation is used when many workers are needed to carry out an activity. Its use is relatively limited in modern organizations, but it was traditional in early societies, such as tribes, clans, and armies. Organizing by sheer number may be used in such activities as house-to-house soliciting campaigns and membership drives. Unskilled labor crews may be organized in this pattern.

Orphan Activities

Certain activities may not merit grouping into a separate department, and there may be no compelling reason to place them in any specific location in the organization. Yet, these orphan activities must be coordinated and interlocked with all others. The "most use" criterion is followed to resolve the question of organizational placement. The major department that uses or needs the service most frequently absorbs the activity. Other units that need the service obtain it from the major department to which the activity has been assigned.

Patient transportation in a hospital involves such a set of activities. These services are used by the physical therapy, occupational therapy, radiology, and other departments, but overall coordination is assigned to the inpatient nursing units because one central placement is needed for these groups of workers. Another example can be seen in the small nursing home where one worker performs several activities on a limited basis, such as general maintenance, messenger and errand service, and transport of patients to appointments with private physicians. The individual with these responsibilities may report to a central manager, such as the director of nursing, since the director or a delegate is present on all shifts. This arrangement provides coordination and control of the activities.

Deadly Parallel Arrangements

In an alternative organizational pattern, the higher levels of management establish dual organizational units for the purposes of control and/or competition. As a control device, the parallel arrangement permits comparison of costs, productivity, and similar parameters. Competition may be enhanced, if this is desired as a means of motivation, because productivity and performance can be compared.

FLEXIBILITY IN ORGANIZATIONAL STRUCTURE

Managers, in their role as change agents, continually seek ways to respond to change in the external and internal organizational environment. It may be necessary to adjust traditional organizational patterns because of advances in modern technology, the increase in workers' technical and professional training, the need to offset employee alienation, and the need to overcome the problems inherent in decentralized, widely dispersed units.

The classic patterns of organizational structure have included the predominance of functional departmentation with strong emphasis on unity of command. When technical advice or assistance was needed, staff roles were developed to assist the line managers. When interorganizational communication and cooperation among several units were needed, the committee structure was employed. Three alternative temporary or permanent organizational patterns allow managers to retain the benefits of these traditional practices and to reduce some of their disadvantages: (1) the matrix approach, (2) temporary departmentation, and (3) the task force (see Chapter 6). These approaches may supplement the traditional organizational structure or, in the case of the matrix approach, supplant it.

Matrix Organization

Matrix organization, a design that involves both functional and product departmentation, is used predominantly to provide flexible and adaptable organizational structure for specific projects in, for example, research, engineering, or product development. This pattern is also called the grid or lattice work organization and project or product management. The matrix of organizational relationships involves a chief for the technical aspects, an administrative officer for the managerial aspects, and a project coordinator as the final authority. This dual authority structure is a predominant characteristic of the matrix organization and stands in distinct contrast to the unity of command in the traditional organizational pattern.

Workers essentially are borrowed from functional units and given temporary assignments to the project unit. Rather than designating line and staff interactions, the developers of the matrix pattern seek to create a web of relationships among technical and managerial workers. Multiple reporting systems are developed and communication lines are interwoven throughout the matrix.

Participants in the matrix organizational pattern tend to be highly trained, self-motivating individuals with a relatively independent mode of working. These functional personnel are grouped together according to the needs dictated by the phase of the project that has been undertaken. In the matrix arrangement, workers receive direction from the technical or the administrative chief as appropriate, but it is assumed that they have the ability to develop the necessary communication and work patterns without specific direction in every aspect. The project coordinator has the traditional responsibilities of guiding the technical and administrative groups and of developing the basic channels of communication and lines of coordination; however, there may be none of the detailed stipulations that are commonly associated with the highly bureaucratic traditional organizational pattern. In the health care organization, a matrix organization frees nurses, physical therapists, occupational therapists, and other direct patient care professionals from some of the relatively rigid elements of formal organization.

Temporary Departmentation

The temporary department or unit reflects a management decision to create an organizational division with a predetermined lifetime to meet some temporary need. This lifetime may be imposed by an inherent, self-limiting element, such as funding through a defense contract or private research grant. Although the predominant organizational structure may be modified periodically, there is an implicit assumption that the basic unit will remain substantially unchanged for the life of the organization. The use of the term *temporary* may be somewhat misleading: temporary departmentation usually reflects an organizational pattern that will exist for more than a few months, since an activity limited to only a few months' duration would be placed under the category of special project or task force rather than temporary departmentation. Several years may be involved, although there is no set rule.

The development of a new product, i.e., the calculation of comparative cost data, product development, and marketing, may be placed under a temporary department assigned to carry out the necessary research development and marketing within a specific time period. A team of workers with the necessary specialized knowledge may be assembled under the jurisdiction of the temporary department, deadlines set, necessary accounting processes developed, and related functions delineated.

In businesses and institutions with defense contracts or research grants, temporary departmentation provides the necessary organizational structure without interference with the establishment's normal efforts. Equipment is purchased and workers hired with special funds designated for that purpose. These workers are not necessarily subject to the same pay scale, fringe benefits, union contracts, and similar regulations as are regular employees. The manager must make it clear to these workers that their jobs are temporary, limited to the life of the contract or grant. There should also be a clear understanding about worker movement into the main organizational unit: Is this employee eligible for such movement with or without having accrued seniority and similar benefits? Patients who receive full or partial subsidy for their care in a health care institution under a special research grant or project should be informed about the limited scope of the project, and their options for continuity of care after the life of the project should be explained.

THE ORGANIZATION CHART

The management tool for depicting organizational relationships is the organization chart. It is a diagrammatic form, a visual arrangement, that depicts the following aspects of an institution:

1. major functions, usually by departments
2. the respective relationships of functions or departments
3. channels of supervision
4. lines of authority and of communication
5. positions (by job title) within departments or units

There are numerous reasons for using organization charts:

• Since such a chart maps major lines of decision making and of authority, managers can review it to identify any inconsistencies and complexities in the organizational structure. The diagrammatic representation makes it easier to determine and correct these inconsistencies and complexities.

• An organization chart may be used to orient employees, since it shows where each job fits in relation to supervisors and to other jobs in the department. It shows the relationship of the department to the organization as a whole.

• The chart is a useful tool in managerial audit. Managers can review such factors as the span of management, mixed lines of authority, and splintered authority; they can also check that individual job titles are on the chart, so it is clear to whom the employee reports. In addition, managers can compare current practice with the original plan of job assignments to determine if any discrepancies exist.

Certain limitations are inherent in the rather static structure presented by organization charts, and these can offset some of the advantages of their use:

• Only formal lines of authority and communication are shown; important lines of informal communication and significant informal relationships cannot be shown.

- The chart may become obsolete if not updated at least once a year, more frequently if there is a major change in the organizational pattern.

- Individuals without proper training in interpretation may confuse authority relationship with status. Managers whose positions are placed physically higher in the graphic representation may be perceived as having authority over those whose positions are lower on the chart. The emphasis must be placed on the authority relationship and the chain of command.

- The chart cannot be properly interpreted without reference to support information, such as that usually contained in the organizational manual and related job descriptions.

Types of Charts

There are two major kinds of organization charts: master and supplementary. The master chart depicts the entire organization, although not in great detail, and normally shows all departments and major positions of authority. A detailed listing of formal positions or job titles is not given in the master chart, however. The supplementary organization chart depicts a section, department, or unit, including the specific details of its organizational pattern. An organization has as many supplementary charts as it has departments or units.

The supplementary chart of a department usually reflects the master chart and shows the direct chain of command from highest authority to that derived by the department head. The master chart usually shows the major functions, while the supplementary charts depict each individual job title and the number of positions in each section, as well as full-time or part-time status. Additional information, such as cost centers, major codes, or similar identifying information, sometimes appears on the charts.

General Arrangements and Conventions

The conventional organization chart is a line or scalar chart showing each layer of the organization in sequence (Figure 5–3). In another arrangement, the flow of authority may be depicted from left to right, starting with major officials on the extreme left and with each successive division to the right of the preceding unit. The advantage of this form stems from its similarity to normal reading patterns. A circular arrangement in which the authority flows from the center outward is sometimes used; its advantage is that it shows the authority flow reaching out and permeating all levels, not just top to bottom.

Figure 5-3 Master Organization Chart of a Hospital

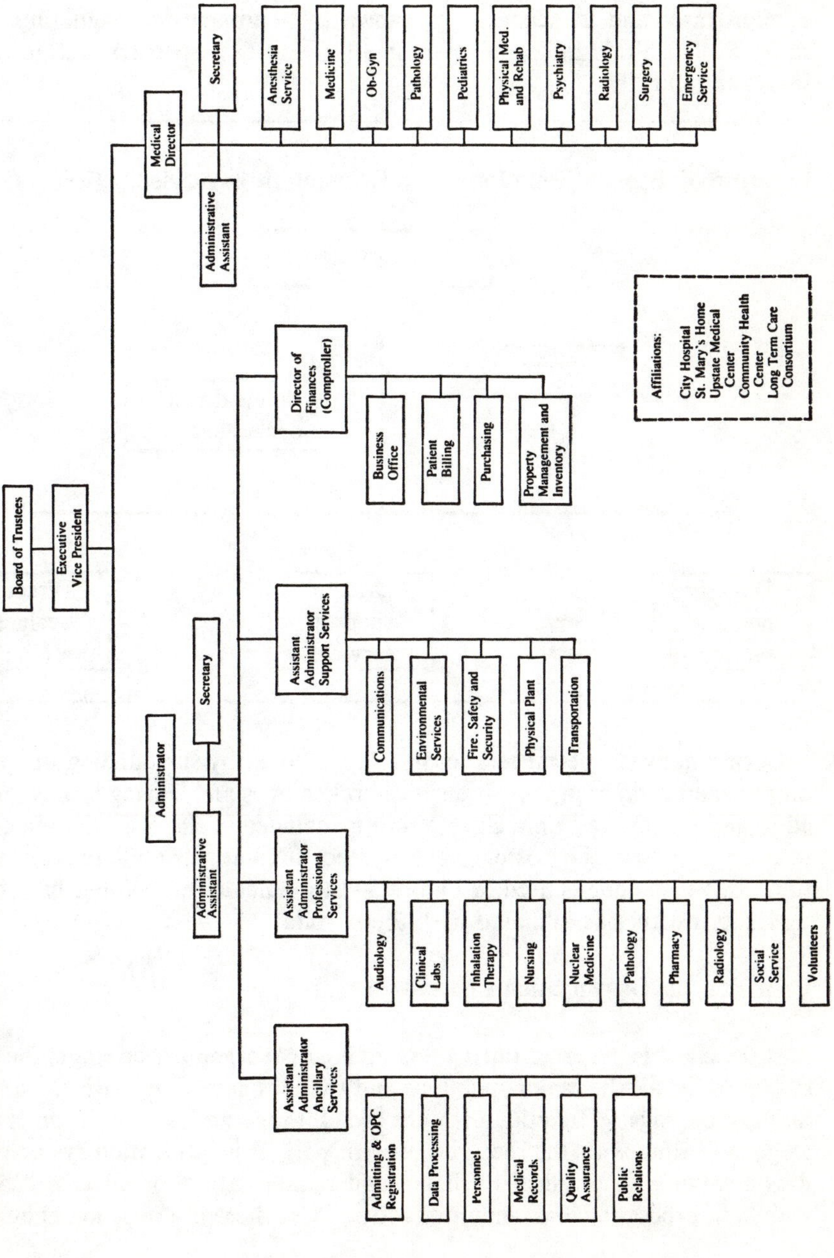

Board of Trustees

Executive Vice President

Administrator

Secretary

Administrative Assistant

Medical Director
- Secretary
- Administrative Assistant
  - Anesthesia Service
  - Medicine
  - Ob-Gyn
  - Pathology
  - Pediatrics
  - Physical Med. and Rehab
  - Psychiatry
  - Radiology
  - Surgery
  - Emergency Service

Director of Finances (Comptroller)
- Business Office
- Patient Billing
- Purchasing
- Property Management and Inventory

Assistant Administrator Support Services
- Communications
- Environmental Services
- Fire, Safety and Security
- Physical Plant
- Transportation

Assistant Administrator Professional Services
- Audiology
- Clinical Labs
- Inhalation Therapy
- Nursing
- Nuclear Medicine
- Pathology
- Pharmacy
- Radiology
- Social Service
- Volunteers

Assistant Administrator Ancillary Services
- Admitting & OPC Registration
- Data Processing
- Personnel
- Medical Records
- Quality Assurance
- Public Relations

Affiliations:
City Hospital
St. Mary's Home
Upstate Medical Center
Community Health Center
Long Term Care Consortium

Certain general conventions are followed when an organization chart is drawn. Ordinarily line authority and line relationships are indicated by solid lines, and staff positions are indicated by broken or dotted lines. In Figure 5–4, the position of medical record consultant has a staff relationship to the administrator and is, accordingly, shown by a broken line. Sometimes the staff relationship is indicated by a small *s* with a slash mark setting it off from the job title:

Figure 5–4 Special Relationships: Consultant in Advisory Role

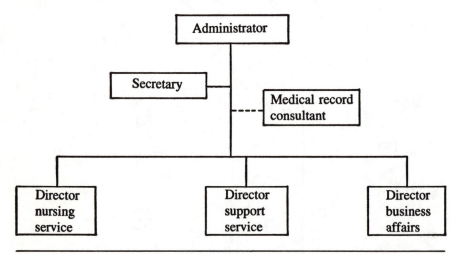

Occasionally, a special relationship is indicated by surrounding an entire unit or even another organization with broken lines and leaving it unconnected to any line or staff unit. Such a unit is included in the organization chart to call attention to the existence of a related, auxiliary, or affiliated organization. This technique is used in Figure 5–3 to indicate the relationship of the teaching institutions affiliated with the hospital.

Preparing the Organization Chart

If the chart is prepared during a planning or reorganization stage, the first step is to list all the major functions and the jobs associated with them. The major groupings by function then are brought together as specific units, e.g., all jobs dealing with the file area or with patient identification systems, all jobs dealing with physical medicine and rehabilitation, or all jobs dealing with data processing and computer activities. If there is a question about the proper placement of one or several functions, managers can derive significant information by asking

- If there is a problem, who must be involved to effect a solution?
- Do the supervisors at each level have the necessary authority delegation to carry out their functions?
- If a change in systems and procedures is needed, who must agree to the changes?
- If critical information must be channeled through the organization, who is responsible for its transmission throughout each unit of the organization?

As an aid in developing the organization chart, it is useful to prepare a simple tabulation showing the following information:

1. job title
2. reporting line: supervised by whom (title)
3. full-time or part-time
4. day, evening, or night shift
5. line or staff position

The inclusion of the incumbent's name is optional for this work sheet preparation, although names may be useful in a subsequent managerial audit of the department in which the manager is comparing present practice with the original plan. The use of names as the basic means of developing the chart could be misleading, however, as it may block managers' thinking, causing them to describe organizational relationships as they are rather than as they should be. It may be best to show names only on a staffing chart that is prepared after the organization chart has been developed.

After obtaining the necessary information about work relationships, shifts, supervisory needs, and span of management factors, managers develop the final chart, using the general conventions for depicting organizational relationships. A support narrative or section of an organization manual can be developed to give additional information.

THE JOB DESCRIPTION

The duties associated with each job should be determined by the needs of the department. Frequently, jobs have evolved as duties have been assigned to an employee, and each job becomes an accumulation of tasks rather than the product of prior planning. Some form of control is necessary to keep assignments within intended limits. In order to provide this control of the various work assignments, the duties and responsibilities of each job should be set forth in written form. This helps to ensure that employees' concepts of their duties will be consistent with those of the manager and with the needs of the department.

In every formal organization, there are job descriptions to cover each job. In order to fill the various positions with the appropriate employees, it is necessary to match the jobs available in the department with the individuals. This can only be done with the help of the job description, a written objective statement defining the content or duties and functions of a job. It includes responsibilities, experience, organizational relationships, working conditions, and other essential factors of a single position.

Job Analysis

The process of preparing a job description is time-consuming, but invaluable. A job analysis must be undertaken in order to collect complete data on the content and requirements of each job so that objective standards can be established. This process may be carried out by the manager, the employee, or consultants. Various methods may be used, including observation, interview, questionnaire, checklists, a daily log, or a combination of these techniques.

When a job analysis is done, the employees must understand that their performance is not being evaluated; it is the job that is being analyzed. Otherwise, the employees may be uncooperative for fear that their jobs will be downgraded with a resultant loss in salary. Each employee should be encouraged to contribute personal thoughts and concerns about the job. Involving the employee is helpful in the collection of data. Everyone should be fully informed of the purpose for the analysis and the methods to be used in the process.

Job Description Format

The format of a job description should present the information in an orderly manner. Since there is no standard format, job descriptions vary with the type of facility, as well as with the size and scope of a department. The following format is suggested as a guide:

- job title. The job should be identified by a title that clarifies the position. The inclusion in the job title of such words as *director, supervisor, senior, staff,* or *clerk* can help to indicate the duties and skill level of the job.

- immediate supervisor. The position and title of the individual should be clearly identified.

- job summary. A short statement of the major activities of the job should include the purpose and scope of the job in specific terms. This section serves principally to identify the job and differentiate the duties that are performed from those of other jobs.

- job duties. The major part of the job description should state what the employee does and how the duties are accomplished. The description of duties should also indicate the degree of supervision received or given.

- job specifications. A written record of minimum hiring requirements for a particular job comes from the job analysis procedure. The items covered in the specifications may be divided into two groups:

1. The skill requirements include the mental and manual skills, plus the personal traits and qualities needed to perform the job effectively:

  - minimum educational requirements

  - licensure or registration requirements

  - experience expressed in objective and quantitative terms, such as years

  - specific knowledge requirements or advanced educational requirements

  - manual skills required in terms of the quality, quantity, or nature of the work to be performed

  - communication skills, both oral and written

2. The physical demands of a job may include the following:

  - physical efforts required to perform a job and the length of time involved in performing a given activity

  - working conditions and general physical environment in which the job is to be performed

  - job hazards and their probability of occurrence

Exhibit 5–1 contains excerpts from a typical job description of a clerical position.

Exhibit 5–1 Excerpts from Typical Job Description: Clerical Position

---

Job Summary

This is a clerical position in the health records service of an acute care facility affiliated with a medical school and a research institution. This full-time, day shift position is under the direct supervision of the Assistant Health Records Administrator; incumbent performs duties with relative independence, referring exceptions to policy and procedure to supervisory personnel with the department.

Job Duties

1. Receives visitors to the department; processes their requests by routing them to appropriate supervisors; assists requestor as needed; schedules appointments.
2. Answers departmental telephones and routes calls or takes messages.
3. Takes dictation from transcribing machine and from rough draft and transcribes according to prescribed format.

Job Specification

1. Fluency in English language, both oral and written expression.
2. Ability to type final copy, from both dictation and handwritten copy, error-free, minimum of 50 words per minute (electric typewriter).
3. Minimum of high school graduation or its equivalent and at least one year of secretarial experience or successful completion of postsecondary secretarial school.

Note flexibility in requirement 3; this fosters a nondiscriminatory approach to hiring, giving flexibility to the manner in which an individual may qualify for the position.

In some institutions, the job specifications are organized as a separate record, because the information is not used for the same purpose as the information contained in the job description. The specifications receive the most usage in connection with the recruitment and selection of employees, since this part of the job description defines the qualifications that are needed to perform the job. Job evaluations and the establishment of different wage and salary schedules are other functions that depend on the data contained in the job specifications.

Uses of Job Description

A job description is used primarily as a basis for employee recruitment and selection, but it is also useful for other purposes:

• to establish a rational basis for job ratings and salary schedules

- to clarify relationships between jobs

- to orient and train new employees to their jobs

- to evaluate job performance and training

- to assign or reassign responsibilities

- to serve as a basis for personnel planning

- to review existing practices in a department

- to determine overall compliance with legal, regulatory, and accrediting mandates

The job description should not be treated as a top secret document. All employees should have access to the file of job descriptions. In this way, all employees can learn the full dimensions of their jobs, how their performance will be evaluated, and what their opportunities are for promotion.

Detailed vs. General Job Description

The amount of detail included in a job description is most often determined by management's intent and use of the description. When a job description is used as a tool in teaching new employees how to do their jobs, a considerable amount of the how and why of the job must be included. When it is used for job evaluation, it may be rather general, with few details about how the work is performed. However, this approach makes it difficult to judge the amount of skill and knowledge required for the job by reading the description. Care must be taken to strike a balance between sufficient detail to convey a sense of the job and too much detail, which gives the impression that, if a task is not specifically mentioned in the job description, the employee need not perform it.

When a single occupation has several job levels, such as staff physical therapist and senior physical therapist, the differences in duties and responsibilities should be clearly discernible from reading the job descriptions and specifications. Exhibit 5–2 presents a comparison of excerpts from the job descriptions of the staff physical therapist and senior physical therapist of a typical amputee team. The senior physical therapist is presumed to have more knowledge and skill, thus the senior therapist's job description includes a duty to supervise the physical therapists assigned to the amputee treatment team and to act as a consultant to the physicians on the amputee service.

Exhibit 5-2 Comparative Job Description Excerpts

Amputee Treatment Team	
Staff Physical Therapist	*Senior Physical Therapist*
• Treats patients . . . assumes full caseload	• Supervises amputee team . . . carries adjusted caseload
• Meets with medical staff to report on patient's progress	• Meets with medical staff of amputee service and acts as a consultant to medical staff

Jobs, like the organizational structure of a hospital, are dynamic in nature. Changes in the size and nature of the organization, the introduction of new equipment, or the employment of new treatment techniques—to mention only a few factors—have a definite influence on the duties and requirements of jobs. Thus, the manager and the employees of a department must review the description of each job on a periodic, regular schedule, at least once a year. The document should be dated when it is first prepared, redated when it is reviewed, and again redated when it is revised. An up-to-date accurate job description is essential when the personnel department recruits applicants for a job or when the manager hires new employees, appraises the performance of existing employees, and attempts to establish an equitable wage and salary pattern within the department.

The entrance of labor unions into health care organizations has added another dimension to the job description; it now becomes a legal document. It is utilized to determine the bargaining unit in which an employee can be placed for the purpose of collective bargaining. It helps to determine any change in the scope of responsibilities of an employee or employees in negotiations of new contracts. It is a valid reference for handling and arbitrating grievances. Because a major function of a job description is to provide facts, figures, and logic, it facilitates the maintenance of a balanced relationship among managers, union representatives, stewards, and employees in the hospital or clinic environment.

Chapter 6

Committees

CHAPTER OBJECTIVES

1. Define committee.
2. Differentiate among committee, plural executive, and task force.
3. Identify the purposes and uses of committees.
4. Recognize the limitations and disadvantages of committee structure.
5. Identify means for improving committee effectiveness.
6. Identify the role and functions of the committee chairperson.[1]
7. Understand the importance of minutes and formal proceedings.

Committees have become a fact of life in modern organizations. The democratic tradition in American society, the committee system's history of success in organizations, and the legal and accrediting authority mandates for such activity contribute to the widespread use of committees in health care organizations. Committee participation is an expected part of the daily routine of the chief of service, department head, or manager. The committee structure complements the overall organizational structure, because it can be used to overcome problems stemming from specialization and departmentation. The weakness of specialization is the potential loss of broad organizational vision on the part of the individual manager; however, coordination of action and assessment of the overall organizational impact of a decision may be facilitated when a committee brings together a number of specialists for organized deliberation.

Health care organizations need committees to help consolidate the dual authority tracks within the medical authority structure and the administrative/support structure. The joint conference committee, consisting of representatives from the medical staff, trustees, and administration, is a common example of this use. Functions of health care organizations typically monitored and assessed by committees include pharmacy and therapeutics, infection control, patient care evaluation, surgical case review, medical records, quality assurance and utilization review. Table 6–1 summarizes typical committee participation by various health care professionals.

THE NATURE OF COMMITTEES

A committee may be defined as a group of persons in an organization who function collectively on an organized basis to perform some administrative activity. A committee is more than an informal group that meets to discuss an issue and share ideas, even if such a group meets regularly. The manager who informally calls together a team of subordinates or other managers to talk over an idea or problem is not dealing with a committee. The emphasis in the committee concept is the creation of a structure that has an organized basis for its activity and interaction and that is accountable for its function. The predominant characteristic of the committee is group deliberation on a recurring basis, done in the context of a specific grant of authority.

Committees may be temporary or permanent. The temporary, or ad hoc, committee is created to deal with one issue, such as the implementation of the problem-oriented medical record or cost containment compliance, and its work is limited to that issue. If the problem assigned to an ad hoc committee becomes a recurring one, it may be handled by an existing committee, the

Table 6–1 Examples of Committee Participation

Department Head	Utilization Review	Medical Records	Risk Management	Quality Assurance
Occupational Therapy	*	*	X	X
Physical Therapy	*	*	X	X
Medical Technology		*	X	X
Dietary		*	X	X
Health Records	*	X	X	X
Nursing	X	X	X	X
Social Service	X	X	*	X

Note: *, rotating membership with other department heads; X, permanent ex officio membership.

issue may be referred to an existing department, or a new standing committee may be created.

Standing committees, which are relatively permanent, focus on recurring matters. The individual members change, but the committee is continuing with respect to the number of members, the distribution of representatives, and its basic charge. Standing committees in health care organizations typically involve credentials, infection control, patient care policies, medical records, and quality assurance. A department may have specific standing committees, such as departmental quality assurance, safety control, or professional development.

A committee may have either line or staff authority. If the committee has authority to bind subordinates who are responsible to it, it is part of the line unit structure. For example, a governing board may have an executive committee that gives directives to the chief executive officer of the institution and thus exercises line authority. A grievance committee, whose decision is binding because of a policy or union contract, exercises line authority in producing its determinations; managers are not free to act contrary to such decisions. If, on the other hand, the committee has an advisory relationship to line managers, it is a staff unit.

In actual practice, the distinction between line and staff authority of a committee is sometimes blurred. A credentials committee of the medical staff may have limited line authority in that, except for unusual cases, the next levels of authority are bound by the recommendations it makes. A union contract governing faculty at a medical school or university may require that a faculty committee review each case of promotion and tenure and make a recommendation to the line officer, the dean, who in turn must add a recommendation, with the final decision made by the board of trustees. Participation in the decision process by several layers in the hierarchy is mandatory in such cases. In that sense, the credentials committee of the medical staff, as well as the promotion and tenure committee of a college, may be viewed as a line committee with limited but explicit input into decisions concerning professional colleagues. Their decisions are not final, but their recommendations are well protected by custom and, in some cases, by law.

The Plural Executive

Although most committees are nonmanagerial in nature, there is a structural variation in which a committee is created that has line authority and undertakes some or all of the traditional functions of a manager. These committees are created as a result of policy decisions. A familiar example in the health care setting is the executive board of a national professional association. Established through the bylaws of the organization, the executive board typically consists of the elected officers and has the authority to act on behalf of the membership in prescribed areas. The board of trustees in a hospital is also a plural executive, although it is almost universal practice to appoint a chief executive officer and assign management functions to that officer.

The plural executive may be established by law, as in federal regulatory agencies (e.g., the Federal Communications Commission and the Securities and Exchange Commission) or in special federal agencies (e.g., the Tennessee Valley Authority). The law creating such agencies stipulates that there be a regulatory board (usually) of 5 to 11 members who have line authority as a board. The board varies greatly in the amount of power held and authority exercised. Although the board has formal authority, the center of true power in the organization may shift from the executive board to the appointed chief executive officer, who reports to the executive board.

The individual officeholders who constitute the plural executive must rely greatly on an appointed officer, such as the executive director, and on the staff chosen by that officer. While the executive officer is in a continuing position, the plural executive group may meet infrequently, and its membership may change as frequently as every year. Furthermore, the members of the plural executive unit tend to remain less visible, as they give directives to the executive, who issues these under the office's title. This common practice often obscures the authority constellation proper to the plural executive and may even reduce it to one of symbolic rather than actual authority and power.

The Task Force

A temporary organizational unit, the task force is created to carry out a specific project or assignment and present its findings to line authority. It has as its focus highly specific work that requires technical expertise. The task force analyzes the question, completes the research, and makes its recommendations, which may take the form of a complete plan of action. Unlike committees, which remain in existence until specifically dissolved, the task force automatically ceases functioning when its assigned task is completed.

Members of a task force are chosen on the basis of technical competence and specialized training to form a composite, interdisciplinary team. They are not selected to represent a special group interest, and not every department or organizational unit is represented. A task force rarely, if ever, has line authority. Its findings sometimes are referred to a committee that deliberates issues of a basic policy nature; the work of the task force complements that of committees by providing technical research and preparing background information. The group may be created as a result of committee deliberations; for example, the executive committee or the board of trustees of a health care institution may wish to expand its services or to develop an entirely new physical complex. These technical problems could be referred to a task force for study; when the work of the task force is done, the line authority takes appropriate action.

A task force sometimes is created for its symbolic value—a common political use. The various presidential commissions of the last decades are examples of the use of task forces to call attention to an important issue, e.g., civil rights, space technology, and care of the aged. In order to provide an arena that is relatively free from vested interests and particular biases, a task force rather than administrative agency or department personnel may be assigned the responsibility of studying the issue.

THE PURPOSES AND USES OF COMMITTEES

Committees are created to fulfill various specific needs. The following purposes and uses of committees include the advantages that accrue to an organization as a result of effective committee structure development.

To Gain the Advantage of Group Deliberation

Many management problems are so complex that their impact on the organization as a whole is best assessed through group deliberation and judgment. Decisions may have a long-range effect, and no single manager has the knowledge necessary to see all the ramifications of a problem. In a committee structure, no one manager bears the burden of a decision that is far-reaching in organizational time and space. Probing of the facts and their implications is likely to be more thorough, as the cumulative knowledge, experience, and judgments of several individuals are brought to bear on the problem in a coordinated manner. The stimulation of shared thinking may lead to a better decision than could be reached by an individual. Finally, group deliberations may be mandatory in some organizations because of the stipulations in a union contract, an accrediting agency, or a regulatory body.

To Offset Decentralization and Consolidate Authority

In the process of organizing, each manager is given only a portion of the organization's authority. Normally, each manager receives sufficient authority to carry out the responsibilities of the branch or unit of the organization over which that individual has charge. When the organizational structure is consolidated, efforts are made to avoid splintered authority. Yet, because of the limits placed on the manager's authority, not every problem a manager faces can be solved nor every plan implemented. It is necessary to consolidate organizational authority through specific coordinating efforts, and committees provide an additional organizational structure that can be used for this purpose.

The creation of a special purpose committee to deal with a project or problem involving several units of an institution is an acceptable means of augmenting the normal organizational structure. Should the problem be a recurring one, the structure itself should be adjusted to consolidate authority in a formal manner through department structure. For nonrecurring special problems, however, the special purpose committee is appropriate.

Coordination among units in a highly decentralized organization may be fostered through committees. The focus under these circumstances is the need for consistency of action and coordination of detailed plans among several units, which are often separated geographically. The Health Systems Agency and the statewide Health Coordinating Committee in health care planning are examples of committees created specifically for the purpose of coordinating activity among units with wide geographical distribution and multiple categories of membership.

To Counterbalance Authority

The check and balance system in an organization is subject to many pressures. When individuals in decentralized locations surrender authority to successive levels in the hierarchy, there is an attendant desire to monitor those higher levels. For example, in order to avoid a concentration of power in an executive director, a professional organization or a union with nationwide membership may create an executive committee with power to finalize all decisions, to approve the budget and authorize payments over a stated amount, and to act as sole decision-making body in many areas.

In a situation in which there has been significant fraud, deception, or extreme authoritarianism, an officer may be retained temporarily to avoid a public scandal that would have negative effects for the organization. To limit the actions of such an individual during the transition period, the authority of the office is stripped away and placed in a special group that acts as a line committee in place of the official, who retains only the title and selected symbols of office. This committee functions until the officer is safely removed in a politically acceptable manner and a successor is chosen. The committee structure can be costly in economic terms, but an organization may be willing to pay the price to offset concentrated power and to obtain a diffused authority pattern in certain circumstances.

To Provide Representation of Interest Groups

Occasionally, certain groups have a vested interest in an organization and seek representation in its decision-making arenas, including committee participation. Wanting to protect the value of their degrees, alumni of a college seek positions on the board of trustees or on advisory committees to specific programs. Community members concerned with both long- and short-range plans of a health care organization seek input into patient care policies and community health programs through committee participation.

The organization, in turn, is interested in obtaining the support of specific groups and extends to them an opportunity to participate in its deliberations, often through the committee structure. A college may seek alumni representation to consolidate financial support from that group. A hospital or health center may seek community representatives for its advisory committee, the better to determine local sentiment, assess probable response to changes in the pattern of services offered, and to gain tangible financial support and the more intangible fund of good will toward the institution.

To Protect Due Process

In disciplinary matters, an organization may seek to reflect the larger societal value of due process, even when there is no legal or contractual requirement to do so. An increase in litigation has added an almost legal flavor to processes in which an individual's performance is evaluated. A committee of the individual's peers, even if the peer group does not have line authority, may be constituted to make a recommendation to the line officer or governing board. Examples of this approach include the promotion and tenure committee of a university, the ethics committee of a professional association, or the credentials committee of a medical staff. A union contract may specify the composition and function of a grievance committee to ensure that it includes line workers as well as management officials.

To Promote Coordination and Cooperation

When individuals affected by a decision have participated in making that decision, they are more likely to accept it and abide by it. Participants in group deliberations develop a fuller understanding of each unit's role. The communication process is facilitated, since the managers affected by the decision have had an opportunity to present their positions, the constraints under which their departments function, and their special needs, as well as to express disagreements. All members can evaluate the overall plan, review their own functions, and become familiar with the tasks assigned to other units that depend on their unit's output or, in turn, constrain the work assigned to their unit. In its final decision or recommendation, the committee states the assignments for each unit, and these are known to all. This is especially valuable when the success of the work depends on the full understanding and acceptance of the decision and plan of execution.

To Avoid Action

A manager who wishes to avoid or postpone an action indefinitely may create a committee to study the question or may refer it to a panel that has a long agenda and sends its findings to yet another committee for action. If members are selected carefully or if the assignment to an existing committee is made strategically, action will be slow. The issue may die for lack of interest or may become moot because of a decision made in some other arena or because of the departure from the organization of the individuals concerned. Although this intentional delaying tactic can be misused by a manager, it may also be a positive strategy; for example, delay through committee deliberation may be a form of "buying" time for issues to become less emotionally charged.

To Train Members

Committee participation may be used as part of the executive training process. Exposure to multiple facets of a decision, the defense of various positions, and the development of insight into the problems and considerations of other managers' decisions are part of this training experience. The potential manager is assessed by other members of the executive team during this interaction, and appropriate coaching and counseling may be given to the management trainee.

LIMITATIONS AND DISADVANTAGES OF COMMITTEES

Humorous and disparaging comments sometimes reflect the limitations and disadvantages of committee use: "A camel is a horse that was designed by a committee." or "There are no great individuals in this organization, only great committees."

Committee interaction, with its emphasis on deliberation and group participation, is slow. The committee structure, therefore, is not the proper arena for making decisions that must be made quickly. The time consumed, including the hours spent in formal meetings, is also costly. In highly decentralized organizations or professional associations, travel and lodging costs alone may run as high as $3,000 for a meeting of only a few members. The cost of an individual member's attendance (separate from travel and related costs) is calculated by establishing an average hourly rate per member and multiplying the meeting time by this rate. For example, an executive committee in which ten department heads participate meets a minimum of 2½ hours once a week. Their salaries are calculated and an hourly rate obtained. At an average of $20 per hour per member, a typical meeting of such a group costs at least $500, not including preparation, follow-up time, or the cost of staff support and services. The results of committee action should offset the costs in time, money, and overall effort.

Because of time pressures, committee deliberations may be cut short, thus removing the major advantages of the committee structure, i.e., group participation and presentation of multiple viewpoints. The committee may be indecisive because there is insufficient time to deliberate, or the discussion may become vague and tangential, leading to adjournment without action. Members' lack of preparation prevents full discussion of issues. Being present and on time is only part of a committee member's responsibility; member preparation is a critical factor.

There are several pitfalls to be avoided in regard to preparation. Material may be prepared and distributed in a timely manner, but the committee members may fail to brief themselves prior to the meeting. A member of a subcommittee may fail to carry out an assignment that is critical for the panel's further action. Staff aides or the chairman may be late in preparing items so that committee members arrive to find large quantities of critical material at their places and are expected to reach decisions without the time to develop an informed opinion.

Members' absenteeism or tardiness may obstruct the committee's work. If a quorum is required, absence or lateness (or early departure) may upset the critical balance. If the discussion of an agenda item is dependent on a particular member's presence, this part of the meeting must be delayed or postponed if that member is absent or late. Furthermore, time spent waiting for members to arrive to provide a quorum or to discuss a particular agenda item generates cost with no offsetting productivity.

Obstructionist behavior in committee meetings can limit debate. On the one hand, a member who continually declines to give an opinion and who continually votes "abstain" muddies the outcome. The committee may be seen as lacking in decisiveness, and its recommendations may be set aside more easily. On the other hand, an individual or a few members may try to dominate the committee. When unanimity or at least major consensus is required, such members may refuse to give in or may insist on their own suggestions for compromise. The committee, in order to act, must accept this dominance by a few. A ready solution to this problem is the encouragement of minority reports. Some open discussion of group dynamics may also foster solutions to this type of roadblock.

Even with much good will and a high degree of commitment on the part of members, certain aspects of committee dynamics tend to limit the group's effectiveness. In seeking common ground for agreement and in dealing with small group pressures to be polite and maintain mutual respect, diluted decisions or compromise to the point of least common denominator may characterize committee decisions.

Furthermore, a committee never can take the place of individual managers who accept specific responsibilities and exhibit leadership that is a personal, not a group, trait. Managers must accept the responsibility for certain decisions, even when they are unpopular. It may be especially important to have a specific individual held responsible for decisions in conflict situations. The proverbial buck stops at the highest level of officers, and one manager must be the first among equals when it is a decision in that manager's area of jurisdiction.

ENHANCEMENT OF COMMITTEE EFFECTIVENESS

Committees, in spite of their limitations, are valuable for organizational deliberations. Their effectiveness may be enhanced in several ways:

- viewing committee activity as important and legitimate
- providing the necessary logistical support
- assigning clear-cut responsibility and specific functions to the committee
- considering committee size, composition, and selection of members carefully
- selecting the committee chairmanship carefully
- maintaining adequate documentation and follow-up activity
- creating a task force as an alternative to the proliferation of committees
- ensuring that members are sensitive to group dynamics and organizational conflict

Legitimization of Committee Activity

Top management of an organization must create a climate in which the work of committee members is valued. The evaluation system for merit raises and promotions should include the assessment of individuals' work on committee assignments. Committee membership should be viewed positively by members rather than merely tolerated as a duty. Job descriptions should include committee assignment as a necessary component of the work. When staffing patterns are established, work hours should be allotted for essential committee participation. Committee structure should be streamlined so that action is purposeful and members can see the results of their work. Training specifically for effective committee involvement should be part of the overall training program for members, rather than left to chance.

Logistical Support

All necessary staff assistance should be given to the committee chairperson and members. Staff assistants may prepare specific material, research questions, gather necessary support data, and carry out follow-up activities. Clerical support should be provided for recording and transcribing minutes and related documents. Adequate space is made available for meetings. Top management may enhance committee workings by requiring that committee meetings be scheduled regularly and that membership be drawn from several organizational components. Setting aside a certain block of time for interdepartmental meetings and proscribing intradepartmental sessions during that period facilitates the coordination of schedules. If it is deemed preferable, committee meetings may be scheduled for longer periods of time at less frequent intervals.

Clear Scope, Function, and Authority

When a committee is created, its purpose and function, as well as its scope of activity, must be presented clearly. Will its purpose be merely to deliberate? Will it deliberate and make a recommendation, or will its decision be a binding one? What subjects will it consider? For example, will the medical care evaluation committee concern itself only with assessments of the topics of quality assurance that are mandated by outside review agencies, or will it expand its function to organization-wide quality assurance and education? Will utilization review remain a separate function? Will the medical record committee focus only on the records of inpatients or on the medical records of all patients who receive care in the institution, regardless of patient category (e.g., inpatient, outpatient, group practice).

The scope of the committee's work is shaped by its authority. If the credentials committee of the medical staff only makes recommendations to the governing board, while the board retains final authority to make staff appointments, this should be stated in the bylaws creating the panel and setting forth its mandates. The committee's accountability also needs delineation. To whom does it make its reports? How frequently? Is coordination required with certain administrative components or with other committees?

Committee Size and Composition

No absolute figure can be given as the optimum size of a committee. Since open, free deliberation is a major reason for a committee, the size of the group should be small enough to permit discussion. On the other hand, it should be large enough to represent various interest groups. The organization's bylaws and charter may stipulate required committee composition, which, in turn, will affect the group's size. Some hospital policies, for example, state that all chiefs of service are members of the executive committee; therefore the size of the committee is determined by the organization's department structure.

The need for a quorum to undertake official committee action presents special problems if members' schedules simply do not allow them to attend meetings on a predictable basis. Committee size may be increased in order to ensure a quorum so that business may be conducted.

Committee composition is one of the most important factors in the success of a group's work. Whether they volunteer, are appointed, or are elected, members should possess certain personal qualities; they should be able

- to express themselves in a group
- to keep to the point
- to discuss issues in a practical rather than theoretical way
- to give information that advances the thinking of the group about the topic rather than about themselves
- to assess a topic in an orderly yet flexible way
- to suppress the natural desire to speak for the sake of being heard or of saying what they think the leader or some powerful member wants to hear

The members also should have sufficient authority to commit the unit or group that they represent to the course of action adopted by the committee. If an individual is appointed to a committee to represent a busy executive, that person should have the power to cast a vote that binds the executive who deputized the member. Deputizing is not without its hazards, but they may be avoided by careful review and discussion between the executive and the representative before the meeting.

Generally, committee members should be of approximately equal rank and status in the organization in order to permit the free exchange of ideas. The presence of ex officio members, who may be viewed as more powerful than the elected members, may deter free discussion. Individuals who attend meetings as staff assistants should respect the limits placed on their participation. There should be a clear understanding that the duties of secretary of the committee are those of the individual appointed or elected from within the group; another person who is present to carry out the clerical aspect of secretarial work, such as taking down the raw proceedings from which minutes will be extracted, should not be asked to participate in the discussion and should not volunteer information or opinions. If a parliamentarian who is not a member of the committee attends the meeting, this individual should confine any interaction with the committee to points of parliamentary procedure and should withhold all opinions, agreements, and disagreements concerning the issues under discussion. A group that appoints or elects a committee should have confidence that only those individuals duly appointed or elected will make decisions and recommendations on its behalf.

While diverse points of view should be represented in deliberations, not every participant must be a full-time committee member. Individuals can be invited to attend a meeting or a portion of one in order to answer questions from the committee, share information, or present a point of view. Like staff assistants, individuals who attend meetings as guests should respect the limits of their participation.

In summary, committee size and composition are matters of individual organizational determination. Committees should be large enough to represent various interest groups and ensure adequate group deliberations, but small enough so that intragroup deliberation will be effective.

THE COMMITTEE CHAIRPERSON

Committee Chairperson

The position of chairperson of a committee may be filled in several ways. One is direct appointment by the individual with the mandate and the authority to do so. The bylaws of an organization may direct the president of the medical staff to appoint a committee chairperson. The manager of a department may be the chairperson of a related committee as a matter of course: the director of the utilization review program may be the appointed chairperson of the utilization review committee; the individual who holds the line position of safety automatically becomes the chairperson of the safety committee.

Managers may appoint themselves chairpersons of committees that they constitute and over which they wish to exercise control, or they may offset powerful members by appointing as chairperson an individual sympathetic to their position. Selection of committee chairpersons may or may not be left to the group's membership. In committees where members are elected from the panel as a whole and where there is an accepted egalitarianism in the group, this is a common practice. The group conveys the idea that all those selected for membership have equal ability and that equal confidence is placed in all of them. Conversely, the group also could convey the idea that the committee is not very important so it does not matter who is chairperson. A group that elects the members of a committee may select the chairperson as a separate action by a special vote or may direct that the individual who receives the highest number of votes automatically assumes the chairpersonship.

Occasionally, the office is simply rotated among members of the committee in order to avoid a power struggle. When a specific activity of a standing committee requires extensive and recurring follow-up work and staff assistance is limited, the work of the chairperson is divided by rotation; since the burden of staff support must be shared by the chairperson's department or unit, this approach spreads the support work over several organizational units. When the committee's work is viewed as mere compliance with bureaucratic red tape and the work is not valued by its members nor by the group as a whole, the position of chairperson is sometimes downplayed by this rotation process. Finally, individual members may volunteer to accept the assignment as chairperson, either because of a sense of duty or because of a desire to advance personal position, to protect some potentially threatened interest, or to coordinate the work of a committee dealing with an issue within their field of expertise.

An able well-qualified individual sometimes refuses to accept the position of chairperson because it limits ability to participate in deliberations. Eligibility factors sometimes determine the choice of a chairperson. Prerequisites might include prior membership on the committee, tenure as a faculty member, ten years of service as a full-time employee, or a certain technical or professional degree.

A committee chairperson's duties include arranging for logistical support, chairing meetings, and monitoring follow-up assignments. Logistical aspects of these duties include

- coordinating schedules of committee members
- correlating committee activities with work of related committees or departments
- checking for compliance with mandated deadlines and actions
- obtaining meeting space
- issuing meeting notices as to time, date, place, and agenda
- coordinating and distributing support information before meetings
- preparing agenda, including sequencing items to give priority as needed

Chairing the Meeting

The chairperson sets the tone of meetings, controls the agenda to a major extent, guides deliberation on the issues, and provides or denies opportunities for committee members to express themselves. The degree of formality or informality is indicated not only by the manner in which the chairperson conducts the business of the meeting, but also by an explicit statement. At the outset, the chairperson makes known the rules of debate, e.g., whether there will be general discussion followed by a formal vote and whether strict adherence to parliamentary procedures will be required throughout the meeting.

It is the duty of the chairperson to conduct the meeting efficiently by starting the session on time, following the agenda, and providing sufficient time for deliberation. Subtle leadership skills must be brought to bear as the chairperson referees the members' deliberations. The process of group deliberation and participation must be protected and promoted. The chairperson must artfully provide time for individuals to be heard, which is far more than merely letting each person have a turn to speak. Group cohesion must be fostered even when there are differences of opinion.

The agenda is usually prepared by the chairperson. It is intended to guide the proceedings, but the chairperson may take an item out of sequence if the course of discussion creates a natural opening for the deliberation of related agenda items. The chairperson keeps the meeting flowing by moving from one agenda item to another at appropriate times, calling the group's attention to work accomplished and work yet to be done.

The chairperson must seek to prevent polarization, too hasty decisions, or the eruption of blatant conflict. It is the chairperson's duty to prevent the group from moving into discussion of nonrelated topics or returning to issues that have already been settled. The chairperson periodically integrates the discussion by summarizing major points, calling for motions, and appointing subcommittees or individuals to carry out special assignments.

Follow-up Activity

The final duty of the chairperson is follow-up. The chairperson participates in the preparation of minutes either directly by formulating them or indirectly by reviewing and approving them as prepared by the committee secretary. Periodic reports must be made to administrative officials. In addition, the chairperson must write letters to invite special guests, consult technical staff, hold informal sessions with members between meetings, and attend subcommittee meetings or those of related committees; all these fall within the duty of follow-up for proper committee functioning.

The chairperson must periodically review the work of the committee. Is this work satisfying the basic charge to the committee? Is the committee fulfilling its designated function? The minutes of several recent months may be examined and specific follow-up inquiries made to individuals and sub-committees concerning the progress of work assigned; agenda items that were set aside or those not discussed for lack of time should be brought to the committee's attention again. All unfinished business should be monitored. Exhibit 6–1 is a form a committee chairperson may use to facilitate this follow-up. Exhibit 6–2 provides an example of a tabulated form for recording minutes.

MINUTES AND PROCEEDINGS

Sound practice requires that organizations maintain an official documentation of business transacted. Minutes serve as the permanent factual record of committee proceedings. An explicit statement in bylaws or policies may state that the minutes shall be maintained, including record of attendance; that they shall reflect the transactions, conclusions, and recommendations of each meeting adequately; and that they shall be maintained in a permanent file. Some other time frame for retention that reflects the legal and statutory requirements for the organization may be stated. Committee manuals reflect such information.

Properly formulated, minutes summarize business transacted, including matters that require follow-up action, those on which there is substantial agreement or disagreement, and issues that remain open for committee deliberation. Minutes are sometimes transmitted to individuals who are not currently members, as determined by the policies on distribution and by legal and accrediting requirements. The historical record provided in the minutes gives new members an overall sense of committee activity. A surveyor checking for compliance with utilization review requirements may request the minutes of the utilization review committee over the past year. Representatives of the Joint Commission on the Accreditation of Hospitals (JCAH) may call for minutes and proceedings of the medical staff committees to help in determining whether the staff is fulfilling its medicoadministrative responsibilities.

In legal proceedings, the admissibility of committee minutes and proceedings as evidence rests on the premise that these records were made in the normal course of business, at the time of the action or event, and within a reasonable time thereafter. Thus, minutes of official business of the organization's committees must be prepared, reviewed, and distributed in a timely

Exhibit 6–1 Follow-up of Committee Action

Committee _____
Year _____

Agenda Item *Topic*	Meeting Date *Deliberated*	Description	Responsibility *Assigned to*	Next Action *Due*	Date Action *Completed*
Outpatient Clinic Records	May 15	1. Develop chart review list.	Medical Record Administrator	July 20	
Suspension of Privileges for Admitting Patients	June 11	1. Review legal aspects of procedure for suspending physician privileges. 2. Update procedures in light of legal aspects.	Chief of Medical Staff Chief of Medical Staff	July 20 October 17	

Exhibit 6-2 Excerpts from Utilization Review Committee

Date_____

Agency No. Patient Initial	Start of Care	Discharge Date	Findings and Remarks
512-02 F.C.	12/5/82	current	RN, PT, OT: good records; progress documented by all disciplines. RN evaluation had excellent needs assessment and nursing plan. PT evidenced ongoing teaching and good carry over. OT documentation not always legible, but patient progress in ADL was obvious to reviewer. Team cooperation evident throughout record.
513-07 A.B.	1/27/84	current	RN; Aide; ST; OT; PT - No list of medications. Two nursing supervision notes missing; doctors' orders not current. Nursing supervision is evident but aide notes are incomplete. Communication among all disciplines is weak. Why no social service referral? Recommend review of case with all disciplines; needs discharge plan.

manner, close to the time of the actual proceedings. They are reviewed formally at the next meeting to obtain general agreement that their content reflects the business transacted. Should a lawsuit be instituted regarding the possible negligence, malpractice, denial of privileges, or discipline of a practitioner, the minutes of such proceedings might, in some instances, be admissible as legal evidence; the laws on this point vary from state to state.

It could be argued that minutes do not reflect all the business transacted by the committee. The counterargument is a question: Why not? The effort spent on proper documentation in the normal course of business is a legitimate use of organizational time and staff. It has also been argued that minutes could be altered to reflect business that, in fact, was not transacted, but this is true of any form of documentation. Review of minutes by all members is one way to safeguard accuracy. Managers can only go forward guided by their own ethical code as well as by the organizational and societal presumption that the work was carried out "in good faith."

Preparation of Minutes

Minutes are prepared in a two-stage effort. First, the proceedings are transcribed in their entirety by clerical staff, or a summary of key points is compiled by a staff assistant. Then, the official secretary to the committee, if there is such an office, or the committee chairperson, formulates the official minutes from the transcript or summary. If there is no clerical assistant or staff aide, the chairperson (or member-secretary) uses self-compiled notes to formulate the minutes. Any required approval is obtained, and minutes are sent out according to a prescribed distribution list. The distribution process may be simplified by developing a standing list of the names and titles of members, administrative officers to whom certain minutes are sent because of their organizational jurisdiction, and/or the chairpersons of related committees. The chairperson then needs only to check the names of those who are to receive a particular set of minutes. It is useful to include the statement *Standard Distribution* and also to list any additional individuals to whom minutes were sent as a point of information. The inclusion of a list of support material or enclosures makes the minutes more complete.

Exhibit 6–3 illustrates a format that makes it possible to scan the pages of a volume of minutes and focus on specific topics. The topic key should be placed in the right-hand margin; if the left-hand margin is used for the topic key, it may be placed too deeply in a bound or semibound margin for ready reference. Inclusion of the dates on which there was previous discussion gives the user an easy means of reference to related information. This format generates an index of committee topics, and members have the benefit of ready reference to past deliberations of a related nature.

Content of Minutes

Minutes are more than a mere listing of committee actions in chronological order. The topics discussed are normally grouped, a process facilitated by adherence to a formal agenda. In relatively informal meetings, however, the discussion may be diffuse and less focused on discrete topics than is a discussion in a meeting conducted under strict parliamentary procedure.

Exhibit 6–3 Sample Format for Minutes

The committee directed its attention to new guidelines concerning the content of discharge summaries. A random sample of discharge summaries dictated during recent months was compared with the guidelines to determine areas of noncompliance and areas of strength.	DISCHARGE SUMMARIES 7/21/82 9/11/83

The minutes should reflect what is done, not what is said. Adequate minutes as a matter of course contain such information as

- the name of the committee
- the date, time, and place of the meeting
- an indication of whether it is a regular or special meeting
- the names of members present (specify ex officio if appropriate)
- the names of members absent (include a notation of excused absence if appropriate)
- the names of guests, including title or department as an additional indicator of reason for attending

The opening paragraph of minutes, which is relatively standardized, normally includes:

- the name of the presiding officer
- the establishment of quorum, if this is done routinely or at the request of a member
- a routine review of the minutes of the previous meeting, noting whether they were reviewed as read or only as distributed and whether any corrections were made

The proceedings are summarized. The names of those who make formal motions are given, but the names of those who second the motions need not be recorded. All main motions, whether adopted or rejected, are included.

The bulk of the business may be reflected in general discussion only. There are five basic dispositions of agenda items, and each should be listed with its disposition:

1. Item is discussed and a formal motion is made; formal wording of motion is given. Votes for and against, as well as abstentions are recorded. Notation is made whether motion is adopted or rejected.
2. Item is discussed, and there is general consensus. No formal motion is made. Summary statement of general discussion is entered with notation that there was general agreement or assent with action taken.
3. Item is discussed and tabled informally or set aside for discussion at another time because members need more information. Reason for setting it aside may be stated; indeed, it is useful to give this information for later reference.
4. Item is discussed, with subsequent formal motion to table it permanently.

5. Item is not discussed. This is not stated directly; item is simply carried as old business.

A useful practice for providing background information for new members of a committee or for review of past committee action is to include a rationale statement for each motion that is made. Although this is not required, such a statement provides a succinct summary of the underlying reasons for an action:

> It was moved and seconded that chart review will be carried out by medical record department personnel for all patients in the long-term care/rehabilitation unit whose length of stay exceeds 14 days. This review will be made on a weekly basis for each patient.
> *Rationale:* Because of the extended length of stay for this category of patients (an average of 47 days in this facility), the detection and subsequent correction of medical record documentation deficiencies should be carried out during the patients' stay.

Both the positive and negative discussion of each topic may be summarized. If there is a specific follow-up action to be taken and a committee member is assigned this task, the name of the individual should be included in the minutes. If a subcommittee is created, the names of its members are given. In the minutes of a formal meeting, points of order and appeals, whether sustained or lost, are noted.

At the conclusion of the minutes, the name of the individual who compiled them is given. The legend *minutes compiled by* may be used instead of the somewhat archaic phrase *respectfully submitted*. If minutes are approved or reviewed by the chairperson before distribution, this is stated. The minutes should be signed by the person who compiled them (e.g., the committee secretary) and the person who approved them for distribution. If there is no secretary to the committee as a distinct office, the chairperson's name and signature are entered.

NOTE

1. According to strict parliamentarian interpretation, the proper term is *chairman,* with the titles of Madam Chairman or Mister Chairman used as specific indicators; it has become common usage to insert the term *chairperson* in an attempt to avoid nonsexist language.

Chapter 7

Adaptation and Motivation in Organizations

CHAPTER OBJECTIVES

1. Recognize the necessity of integrating the individual into the organization.
2. Identify the techniques that foster integration of the individual into the organization.
3. Identify the patterns of behavior through which workers express their attitude toward the organization.
4. Define the management function of motivation.
5. Identify the theories of motivation.

In order to get work done efficiently and effectively, managers must motivate the worker and assist in the adaptation of the individual to the organizational demands. Individuals must "fit" into the organizational framework. There is a close tie between the motivation/adaptation activities and the controlling function of the manager; the worker who fits the organization and who values an assigned role is likely to be motivated more easily. In turn, the need to control activity, e.g., through disciplinary action, is reduced.

The amount of organizational resources that managers may direct toward controlling the behavior of individuals is limited. Herbert Simon stressed the importance of having the decisions and behavior of individuals influenced by the organization. He observed that the actual physical task of carrying out an organization's objectives falls to the person at the lowest level of the administrative hierarchy.[1] What means of control then are available to managers to shape individual decisions and behavior? Is the primary means of control the system of reward and punishment, or are there other, more diffuse ways in which individuals in society are shaped to accept, with minimal difficulty, the place assigned to them in an organization?

ADAPTATION TO ORGANIZATIONAL LIFE

How do individuals react to the highly bureaucratic structures associated with modern organizations? Are these patterns of accommodation functional or dysfunctional to the individual and to the organization? Two specific factors that result from organizational structure may be cited to illustrate the need for an explicit management process to help integrate the individual into the organization:

1. the need to offset the effect of decentralization
2. the need to coordinate the many individual functions that result from departmentation and specialization

Overall goals and policies for the institution are made at a central level in the hierarchy, and the work is carried out over a wide range of organizational space and time. Occasionally, conflicting directives are issued from central authority. Yet, all functions must be carried out in a stable, predictable, goal-oriented manner.

Two additional factors that stem from the nature of human interaction in organizations should be considered:

1. the sheer number of individuals who enter the organization either as worker/members or as clients
2. the different manner in which individuals react to the complexities of organizational life

These many individuals not only have different values, different personalities, and different life experiences, but also belong to many other organizations, some of which may have values that compete and even conflict with the values embodied in their current workplace. Some of the patterns of accommodation to organizational life may be functional to the organization but dysfunctional to the individual. Potential conflict must be offset, and the personality mixes of workers and clients must be melded into smooth, interpersonal relationships. Again, the need is for work performance that is stable and predictable, regardless of where it is performed or who performs it.

TECHNIQUES TO FOSTER INTEGRATION

Herbert Kaufman analyzed specific techniques used to bring about conformity of action in a large, decentralized organization that sought to preserve individuality and creative thinking:

1. Preformed decisions
   a. authorizations
   b. direction
   c. prohibitions
2. Detecting and discouraging deviation
   a. routine reports
   b. official diaries
   c. inspection
   d. movement of personnel
   e. sanctions
   f. feedback and correction
3. Developing the will and capacity to conform
   a. selection of persons who fit
   b. postentry training
4. Building identification with the organization
   a. transfer and promotion process
   b. use of symbols[2]

In addition to the techniques cited by Kaufman, managers can assess the various aspects of work rules and off-the-job conduct, as well as the impact of the work group and its potential as a force in integrating the individual into the organization.

Preformed Decisions

Events and conditions should be anticipated as fully as possible, and the courses of action to be taken for designated categories of events and conditions should be described. The following are summaries of definitions taken from Kaufman:

1. Authorization: the description of the course of action applicable to any category may be permissive; it may spell out several series of steps among which the employee shall choose. It "permits" an action, guaranteeing that no sanction will be incurred if the action is carried out. It is a grant of power; at the same time, it is a limit on behavior since prohibited action is implied.
2. Prohibition: promulgated to prevent designated actions from arising by establishing penalties for those who commit them. These are explicit limits of power.[3]

These tools of promoting and channeling behavior are both expected and required in any well-managed organization. The policy manual, the procedure manual, the employee handbook, the medical staff bylaws, and the licensure laws for the various health professionals are all routine management tools.

Work Rules

While there is always an implicit understanding of behavior that is accepted or prohibited, certain aspects of work rules are stated explicitly. The statements of rules in an organization may vary from highly specific descriptions of what an individual must or must not do to more general descriptions of what behavior is preferred and/or permitted but not desirable.

Rule formulation generally has been accepted as a management prerogative in the control function. Even in unionized settings, the employee is clearly not a free agent. Collective bargaining agreements frequently include work rule clauses. Work rules extend beyond the behavior of the individual during the paid working hours to include arrival and departure time, breaks and lunches, and, in some circumstances, off-the-job conduct. Work rules are related to motivational processes because they contribute to a stable organizational environment. They serve several functions in an organization:

- to create an overall order and discipline so that members' behavior is goal-oriented
- to help unify the organization by channeling and limiting behavior
- to give members confidence that the behavior of other members will be predictable and uniform
- to make behavior routine so that managers are free to give attention to nonroutine problems
- to prevent harm, discomfort, and annoyance to clients
- to help ensure compliance with legislation that affects the institution as a whole

The organization has a positive duty to protect both clients and workers in health, sanitation, and safety. In addition, it seeks to prevent behavior that has the potential of alienating or offending clients. Because they deal with patients and their families in stress situations, health care organizations have specific obligations in this area.

Rules of behavior in the organization are derived from several sources. The institution may state its acceptance or rejection of certain values of the larger society. It may cite its own philosophical stance. Members entering the organization are expected to accept the organization's philosophy, at least during working hours.

Individuals choose to enter highly normative organizations because they espouse a similar philosophy. The values of a sponsoring fraternal, philanthropic, or religious group are reflected in the work rules of a health care organization under such sponsorship. Behavior acceptable in one organization may not be acceptable in another. Members of professional associations who become members of another organization bring the values and explicit code of ethics of the associations into the organization's values.

Legislation and regulatory directives, such as those prohibiting certain actions by licensed health care practitioners, are other sources of rules. The net effect of rule codification is behavior that is relatively predictable and stable and that distinguishes individuals' conduct as members of an organization from their behavior outside the institution.

Detection and Discouragement of Deviation

Several direct and aboveboard methods to detect and discourage deviation are available to managers. The methods described by Kaufman are positive, methodological means of encouraging compliance through routine, nonthreatening processes that pervade the entire manager-worker interaction. Kaufman cites the use of routine reports, official diaries, inspections, and workload planning as common processes that enable central management to detect deviation from prescribed action.[4]

Reports and Inspections

When reporting and inspection processes are routine, members of the organization are discouraged indirectly from deviation from prescribed methods of performance because their variances are likely to be uncovered. Routine reports and official diaries are maintained in a uniform manner; the specific information to be entered, the format, the period covered, and the date to be filed are mandated. Kaufman noted that problems with falsification of entries tend to be minimal because discrepancies can be noted from one report to another.[5] For example, any discrepancy in reporting an incident in patient care is easily recognized because there are several review levels of the incident documentation.

There are several points at which a medication error must be documented, with several subsequent independent reviews. Key points are the entry on the medication sheet, the pharmacy inventory, the incident report, the nurses' notes in the patient chart, the entry by the physician, risk management chart analysis reporting forms, and medical audit data. Because the information is entered from different perspectives, at different times, for different purposes, it becomes difficult for any one person to falsify it. The routine processes not only encourage factual reporting, but also offer protection to the individual who inadvertently makes an error.

Inspection is another means of management control. Kaufman noted that several inspections, such as fiscal review, safety checks, and general function review, are performed at different times, by different individuals, with different points of focus.[6] Although many people in health care circles feel that the number and kinds of inspections by accrediting and regulatory agencies should be reduced, management would have to spend time and money to create workable audit processes that would have the same effect if it were not for this cycle of required, outside review.

Whether one subscribes to the more military view that what is not inspected deteriorates or whether one approaches the organizational dynamic by the systems concept of entropy (i.e., all organisms have the capacity for maximum disorder or disintegration unless specific efforts are made to overcome this state), the need to detect and discourage deviation must be recognized. A properly constructed control system, with several reporting and inspecting points, serves the purpose of detecting deviation so that it can be corrected; on the positive side, it encourages compliance.

Lateral Movement of Personnel

Kaufman noted that the lateral movement of personnel throughout an organization fostered identification with the organization and, as an unintended but positive effect, discouraged deviation from prescribed practice. With routine movement from one work assignment to another, including shifts in geographical locations, individual forest rangers found steady compliance was the easiest way to avoid difficulty. Their successors would see where there had been a deviation from prescribed practice, not because of one individual's intentional reporting on another, but because of requests for funds, additional personnel, and authorization of overtime or related needs to remedy the faulty situation. All of this is done within a value system that emphasizes honesty and under circumstances in which there is a relatively high identification with the organization.[7]

Lateral movement of personnel is a common practice in several types of organizations. Religious orders, the military, banking and securities firms, and certain large business firms routinely move their members to make them dependent on the organization and to foster identity with the institution as a whole because the unchanging feature in the person's life is the work. In addition, the individual must rely on the procedures and routines that remain the constants in an otherwise changed working environment. When such lateral movement may come at any time, the effect is a continual state of readiness that is conducive to continual compliance.

This concept applies to the health care organization in a slightly different way. The practice of the "float" assignment is usually developed to satisfy the immediate needs of staff fluctuations. A nurse, for example, is moved from one service to fill in, often without prior notice, where there is a pressing need. This nurse must rely more on the accepted professional practices than on individual style or work group style. Rotating shifts have the same effect; it is the work that remains the same, not the team of personal friends.

For several health care professions, the professional world is relatively closed. Although individual practitioners may not belong to a multicomponent organization within which they may be moved involuntarily, there is a kind of voluntary lateral movement inside professional circles, either in a geographical region or in the entire profession. Compliance with accepted professional practice becomes part of the individual's professional reputation, as the practitioner's successor readily sees the areas where there was compliance as well as any deviation from accepted practice. As with the forest ranger, compliance is the safer and easier route.

Sanctions

Both positive and negative sanctions can be used to induce compliance. Bonus pay, merit increases, and special time off with pay are positive sanctions, a kind of reward system; demotion, suspension, and written reprimand are negative sanctions. An essential element in any sanction system is the development of adequate feedback mechanisms and correction where needed. Employee evaluation and training processes also serve this purpose on a routine basis.

Development of the Will and Capacity To Conform

Kaufman stressed two aspects of integrating individuals into the organization that affect the development of the will and capacity to conform. The first of these occurs before the individual becomes a member of the organization; the second involves postentry training. Kaufman defined the first process as selecting people who fit.[8] The more selective an organization is, the more effective the involvement of the members tends to be; their commitment to organizational values is deeper, and they need fewer external controls.

In recruiting members, the highly selective organization appeals to an anticipated audience, composed of individuals who are disposed toward the values of the organization, even at this preselection stage. The selection process may even include the member's family. The situation of the corporate wife or the proscriptions and prescriptions of behavior for the diplomat's family are well-known factors. Recruitment information may emphasize the hardships and difficulties, as well as the positive benefits, or it may include implicit or explicit information about the need to conform.

The authority structure, the nature of the organization, is significant in this regard. The more coercive the organization, the less selective it tends to be. By its nature, the coercive organization accepts as members individuals who do not even want to be a part of it. Organizations tend to be selective and use a highly structured selection process, such as the interview, tests, and probationary periods, in order to choose members who fit. Highly normative organizations vary in their selectivity; some accept almost anyone who wishes to become a member, while others have extensive criteria that must be met prior to acceptance, followed by extensive postentry probation. The contrast in selectivity can be observed in the following situations: draftee or enlistee in the infantry versus officer candidate school; an open admissions process in a publicly funded college versus selective admission to a private college; voter registration drives in widely known political parties versus acceptance as a true adherent to Communist Party affiliation; church affiliation through simple, unofficial attendance at worship services versus six to seven years' probation to make final profession as a member of a religious order.

Kaufman noted that highly structured postentry training is intended to intensify both technical readiness and ability to conform.[9] During this time, new members' technical skills are modified so that they will perform the work according to the specific procedures unique to the organization. Similar processes have been developed in hospitals where professionally trained individuals, e.g., registered nurses, medical record practitioners, and medical technologists, are given special postentry training to familiarize them with the routines of the particular hospital. Businesses use the rotating management internship to foster integration of newly graduated management majors into the organization.

Identification with the Organization

The process of developing strong identification with the organization is enhanced by the internal transfer and promotion process, which adds to the development, adjustment, and broadening of personnel.[10] Beyond this, and perhaps more important, is the effect on the individual. Any continuity, any structure to the person's otherwise fluid work is provided by the organization. The sense of belonging, then, is enhanced; the organization is the major source of personal identity. Through the promotion process, a stable career path may be developed.

Identification with the organization also is fostered through the use of symbols that serve as a common reference point. According to Kaufman,

1. symbols identify the individual as a member of the organization.
2. symbols differentiate the wearer from all others.
3. symbols serve as a link among members.
4. symbols help establish authority and status at a glance.
5. symbols keep individuals aware of their membership and encourage them to think in terms of the organization.
6. symbols provide constant reinforcement of the organization's values so that, in time, its premises become those of the individual.[11]

In addition to providing a mutual frame of reference, symbols are a source of status. They are accepted in the extraorganizational world as an indication of a person's involvement with a particular institution, and they invest that person with the prestige associated with the organization or profession.

Symbols often employed by organizations and associations include badges and uniforms, a motto, a pledge, a code of ethics, or a pin and guard. Titles and even change of personal name are symbolic means of reinforcing organizational identity. Symbolic rewards may be falsified or cheapened by both subtle and overt marketing techniques, yet this desire to have certain symbols indirectly reflects their value. For example, one can purchase a fancy diploma or obscure degree—all with the hope of being identified with the status represented by the symbol.

The hierarchical division, the role and status system, and the specialization and division of labor in health care organizations frequently are reinforced through accepted symbols. A glance at a nurse's cap shows the knowledgeable observer the program from which the nurse was graduated; this, in turn, gives information about the level of the program—diploma, associate degree, or baccalaureate degree—each with its special emphasis. Insignia attest to the training and attendant licensure and certification requirements that the individual has met. Thus, insignia reveal whether an individual is a licensed practical nurse or a registered nurse, a registered occupational therapist or a certified occupational therapist assistant, a registered record administrator or an accredited record technician. Because their level of training is immediately apparent, individual practitioners are not subject to liability or embarrassment as a consequence of being asked to perform some activity beyond their technical competence or their licensure/certification grant of permission. Clients are also protected.

Sometimes role and status are deemphasized. In a psychiatric institution, for example, there may be an emphasis on creating as "normal" an atmosphere as possible, and professional practitioners may set aside the traditional uniform and wear civilian dress. If anonymity is desirable for a group being escorted outside the facility, civilian attire is indicated also. The symbol is manipulated to enforce a selected aspect of the mutual frame of reference.

Rites and ceremonies symbolically emphasize membership in the organization. The significant points of entry, promotion, and departure from the institution are frequently marked by special rites of passage. A member is initiated, inducted, or sworn in as part of the entry process. Dedication to the organization is recognized periodically, as in five-year or ten-year award ceremonies. When the departure from the institution is a positive event, e.g., retirement, the completion of a successful career with the organization is celebrated. When the separation is a negative event, a special "drumming out" ceremony or excommunication rite may be held to emphasize the expulsion of the individual.

Within bureaucratic structures, certain symbols are commonly used to reinforce the status system, e.g., the size, location, and physical enhancements of office space, such as curtains, desk size and quality, and carpet; the quality of stationery; the assignment of a personal secretary rather than a clerk typist or a typist from a central typing pool; the designation of special eating or lounge areas; and the make of car provided. These explicit symbols convey significant information to members and clients of the organization by reinforcing the hierarchical office structure and depersonalizing the office-holder who derives such status from the role assigned by the organization. The need for a sense of belonging, recognition, and status, as well as similar psychological needs, are met by these symbolic modes of identification and role reinforcement.

The conscious recognition that such status symbols are utilitarian, ego-protecting, and role-reinforcing techniques allows the manager to balance their use. By careful use of these techniques, individuals may be brought into the organization and led to voluntary compliance with only minimal use of negative and punitive measures.

The Work Group

An employee's particular role set is continually reinforced by the work group as a whole. Through the work group, the individual is assimilated into the organization or, from a negative aspect, is prevented from being properly assimilated. In addition to the formal prescriptions of interaction, informal patterns of behavior arise among members of the group. Through the informal group, the individual learns the unwritten rules as well as interpretations of the written rules. The informal organization of the work group also satisfies an essential human need: that of belonging. Nonconformity with group norms could bring about the penalty of expulsion from the unit, which would eliminate a vital source of information and communication, as well as a safe arena in which the individual can air conflicts that stem from the formal organizational role demands.

RESPONSES TO BUREAUCRATIC LIFE

If the individual has been successfully integrated into the organization, a certain behavior pattern may be identified as normal, bureaucratic behavior; this behavior is characterized by acceptance of the specialization and the impersonality of large groups. If an individual is unable to make this adjustment, the person may be said to suffer from "bureausis," according to Victor Thompson.[12] This bureaupathology is manifested in two extremes: the bureaupathic response and the bureautic response. Thompson gave the following characteristics as typical of the bureaupath, who exaggerates the aspects of the bureaucratic structure:

- insistence on following all the rules and formalities of procedure

- decision making based on precedence rather than adaptation of response to a changing situation

- accumulation of many records to prove compliance

- a strong resistance to change

- insistence on the rights of the office to offset personal insecurity

- close supervision of subordinates and cool aloofness with clients.[13]

Thompson described the bureautic as a person who is characterized by personal immaturity that, carried over into the bureaucratic setting, causes the individual to feel alienated and powerless. A bureautic client feels lost in the red tape; a bureautic employee feels helpless and believes that only those with pull get ahead. The bureautic constantly violates the rules or refuses to become familiar with them, thus bringing about organizational chaos. Furthermore, this individual fails to keep the necessary records or follow the procedures, insists on personalizing all relationships, and craves a personal response in every interaction. Such a person is unable to look at the abstract goal and disdains the symbols of the organization as lacking meaning.[14]

Patterns of Accommodation

Individuals adjust to highly organized settings in a variety of ways. Robert Presthus suggested that the bureaucratic situation evokes three types of patterns of accommodation: (1) the upward mobile, (2) the indifferent, and (3) the ambivalent.[15] The following is a summary of the main characteristics of these patterns as developed by Presthus.

The Upward Mobile

An individual who identifies deeply with the organization and derives strength from this involvement is an upward mobile. This strong identification not only evokes a sense of loyalty and affirmation, but also provides a constant point of reference. Because the upward mobile accepts the organization's values, the individual is also able to accept its demand for complete conformity. Presthus noted that this individual can overlook the contradictions between the routine operations of the organization and its official myths. The individual possesses the capacity for action despite conflicting alternatives and aims.

The upward mobile finds the order and security of a bureaucratic career appealing and has a general deference for authority and hierarchical status. Anxious to rise in the hierarchy, the upward mobile avoids controversy that might prejudice any future career opportunities, monopolizes status-rewarding activity, and is a "joiner," a carrier of institutional values. The upward mobile carries the job home at night, even choosing off-the-job activities with an eye toward career advancement.

The Indifferent

Unlike the upward mobile, the indifferent refuses to compete for the organizational rewards. Although alienated by the structural conditions of big organizations, the indifferent has come to terms with the work environment. Presthus noted the use of general psychological withdrawal as a means of reducing such conflict. Such a neutral individual redirects interests toward off-the-job satisfactions. Work is not the indifferent's whole life, and the off-the-job activities of this person are rarely job-related.

The indifferent possesses an uncomplicated view of authority so that neither the rewards nor the sanctions are very compelling. The indifferent has no fear of authority, since this person does not seek anything from authority figures and is not driven by exceptional needs for power and success. Although aware of the majority values, the indifferent escapes personal involvement and views the bureaucratic struggle with detachment. Presthus noted that indifferents are often the most satisfied members of the organization, since their aspirations are based on a realistic appraisal of opportunities.

The Ambivalent

The person who neither rejects the promise of power nor plays the role required to get power in the organization is an ambivalent. This individual has high aspirations, but lacks the interpersonal skills of the upward mobile. The ambivalent does not honor the status system and tends to have difficulty with superiors, who are aware that the relationship is based on formal authority, not on esteem. The ambivalent is often a specialist caught between the world of specialized skills and the organizational hierarchy. The response of the ambivalent to organizational life is dysfunctional to that individual, but functional to a certain extent to the institution in that the ambivalent provides insight into organizational dynamics. The ambivalent is sensitive to change and is a catalytic agent in bringing about change. Presthus noted that, apart from this one functional aspect—that of change agent—the ambivalent is uniquely unsuited to the bureaucratic situation.

Client Response to Bureaucracy

The clients of the organization are as affected by the bureaucratic structure as are the employees/members. Therefore, similar patterns of accommodation may be seen in client response to the bureaucratic setting. These "customers" of the organization develop consistent patterns of interaction with the organization's members, exerting both positive and negative influences on the system.

Client demand itself may be the cause of some red tape. In a health care institution, for example, clients may insist that the service be rendered on a first-come, first-served basis. Special efforts to assess walk-in patients through a triage system may be met with both subtle and overt client resistance. There may be an insistence that no clients receive more than their fair share, as determined by the client group, and the client group may become angry with employees who permit an individual to circumvent the procedures or who fail to enforce the rules.

Blau and Scott reviewed selected behavior traits of clients toward employees in public service organizations.[16] Clients who had dealt with the agency over a long period tended to be aggressive and sometimes had the advantage over a new employee who did not yet know the routines. Resentment was identified as another response, especially when sanctions were enforced. Clients sometimes became subservient when employees assumed the attitude that they were doing the clients a favor by carrying out their legitimate requests. A fourth client response was found to be uncooperativeness, a countering of red tape with red tape, such as an insistence on following all procedures in complete detail.

In some establishments, certain job slots or organizational positions are tacitly reserved for members of some client group or for unofficial representatives of that group; this may be done, for example, to maintain an ethnic balance on a school board or a hospital governing board. The acquiescence on the part of the organization to client demand for a power balance may become so strong that it becomes traditional for client wishes to be a major, although invisible, force in the selection of individuals for certain positions.

THEORIES OF MOTIVATION

On the one hand, the manager seeks to develop a work force that fits the organization; on the other hand, the manager must remain aware of the basic needs of the workers. The art of motivating is built on this recognition of human need. Motivation is the degree of readiness or the desire within an individual to pursue some goal. The function of motivating or actuating refers to the ways in which the manager leads the workers to understand and accept the organizational goals and to contribute effectively to these goals. In motivating or actuating, the manager seeks to increase the zone of acceptance within the individual and attempts to create an organizational environment that enhances the will to work. As self-motivation increases, the need for coercive controls and punishment decreases.

Bases of Motivation

Needs are the internal, felt wants of an individual; they are also referred to as drives and desires. Incentives are external factors that an individual perceives as possible satisfiers of felt needs. For example, hunger is a need; food is the satisfier of the need. A review of management history reveals shifting emphases in the understanding of motivation. Frederick Taylor emphasized the incentive wage, Elton Mayo and F. J. Roethlisberger studied the importance of the work group, and Chris Argyris assigned great importance to the need to integrate the individual into the work group. Three theorists whose work focused primarily on the nature of motivation are Abraham Maslow, Frederick Herzberg, and Douglas McGregor.

Maslow's Hierarchy of Needs

Maslow's theory of motivation is predicated on the premise that every action is motivated by an unsatisfied need. Purposeful behavior is motivated by a multiplicity of interests and motivators and, therefore, varies with circumstances and with individuals. Once a need has been satisfied, another level of need must be appealed to in order to motivate workers—a satisfied need is no longer a motivator. Maslow's hierarchy of needs consists of the following scale (from most basic need to higher level, self-actualizing needs):

1. physiological needs (food, water, air)
2. safety and security (order and stability)
3. belonging and social activity (a place in the group)
4. esteem and status (desire for acceptance, prestige)
5. self-fulfillment (full use of talents, self-actualization)[17]

Herzberg's Two-Factor Theory

Herzberg approached the theory of motivation by identifying two factors or elements that are operative in motivation: satisfiers and dissatisfiers. There are, according to Herzberg, many factors in organizational life that satisfy or dissatisfy, including company policy, supervisors, working conditions, or interpersonal relationships among the work group members. If these are perceived as negative or lacking, they are dissatisfiers. If they are present and perceived as "good," they are satisfiers; they are not motivators, however. Herzberg identifies the following as examples of motivators: opportunity for advancement and promotion, greater responsibility, opportunity for growth, and interesting work. His concept of motivators tends to parallel Maslow's higher needs levels—those of esteem and status, and self-fulfillment.[18]

McGregor's Theory X and Theory Y

McGregor set forth a series of assumptions that compare the traditional view of workers (Theory X) with his own view of industrial behavior (Theory Y). The manager who holds the Theory X view believes that employees have an inherent dislike for work and assumes that they have little ambition, will avoid work if possible, and want security above all else. In contrast, the manager who holds the Theory Y view assumes that work is as natural as play or rest; that the average worker, under the right conditions, seeks to accept responsibility; and that workers will exercise self-direction and self-control in the service of objectives to which they are committed.[19]

Contemporary Emphasis in Motivation

Developed primarily by Japanese managers in the late 1960s and 1970s, Theory Z is a contemporary approach to management and motivation that focuses on increased productivity and job satisfaction among workers. The cultural climate in which this pattern of management developed, that of Japan, emphasizes close linkage of work and the worker's life. The phrase *Theory Z* was coined by William Ouchi, who described in detail the elements of this motivational approach:[20] (1) lifelong career with an organization, (2) group decision making, (3) quality circles to foster worker involvement in decisions and control processes, and (4) lateral movement throughout most of the divisions of the organization. Although this approach to management and the class of workers to whom this theory applies is not universal (not all workers are given the lifelong employment option, notably excluded are women and part-time workers), valuable elements of increasing productivity and motivating workers through participative management are present in this theory of motivation.

NOTES

1. Herbert Simon, *Administrative Behavior* (New York: Macmillan, 1957), pp. 2–3.
2. Herbert Kaufman, *The Forest Ranger: A Study in Administrative Behavior* (Baltimore: The Johns Hopkins University Press, 1967).
3. Ibid., p. 92.
4. Ibid., p. 137.
5. Ibid., p. 126.
6. Ibid., p. 138.
7. Ibid., pp. 127 and 155.
8. Ibid., p. 128.
9. Ibid., p. 170.
10. Ibid., p. 178.
11. Ibid., p. 185.
12. Victor Thompson, *Modern Organization* (New York: Alfred A. Knopf, 1961), p. 153.
13. Ibid., pp. 153–169 passim.
14. Ibid., pp. 170–176 passim.
15. Robert Presthus, *The Organizational Society* (New York: Random House, 1962), pp. 166, 178–226 passim, 286.
16. Peter Blau and W. R. Scott, *Formal Organizations* (San Francisco: Chandler Publishing Co., 1962), p. 81.
17. Abraham Maslow, *Motivation and Personality* (New York: Harper & Row, 1954).
18. Frederick Herzberg et al., *The Motivation to Work* (New York: John Wiley & Sons, 1959).
19. Douglas McGregor, *The Human Side of Enterprise* (New York: McGraw-Hill, 1960).
20. William Ouchi, *Theory Z: How American Business Can Meet the Japanese Challenge* (Reading, MA: Addison-Wesley, 1981).

Chapter 8

Authority, Leadership, and Supervision

CHAPTER OBJECTIVES

1. Differentiate among the terms *power, influence,* and *authority.*
2. Recognize the importance of authority for organizational stability.
3. Identify the sources of power, influence, and authority.
4. Relate the sources of power, influence, and authority to the organizational position of the line manager.
5. Recognize the limits placed on the use of power and authority in organizational settings.
6. Identify the styles of leadership.
7. Identify the relationship of leadership to the supervisory activities of issuing orders and directives, taking disciplinary action, and developing training activities.

The manager gives an order or directive, and there is compliance; why did the employee obey? Is it correct to use the term *obey* to describe this compliance? What bases of authority are operative in superior-subordinate transactions? What are the limits of a manager's authority? What if a particular supervisor is seen as a weak manager? Are there any remedies to problems related to weak or ineffective management leadership? Of what value to the organization is the authority structure? What are the consequences to organizational life if there is not a general, untested compliance most of the time? When such actions of compliance are described, which term is the proper point of reference: power, authority, or influence? Are these terms mutually exclusive or are they synonymous when used in the context of organizational relationships? These questions arise when discussion of authority in organizations is undertaken.

Organizational behavior is controlled behavior, directed toward goal attainment. The authority structure is created to ensure compliance with organizational norms, to suppress spontaneous or random behavior, and to induce purposeful behavior. No matter how the work within the organization is divided; no matter what degree of specialization, departmentation, centralization or decentralization is formalized, there must be some measure of legitimate authority if the organization is to be effective. The concept of formal authority is supported by the two related concepts of power and influence. These concepts may be separated for analytical purposes; in actual practice, however, the three concepts are intertwined.

THE CONCEPT OF POWER

Power is the ability to obtain compliance by means of coercion, to have one's own will carried out despite resistance. Power is force or naked strength; it is a mental hold over another. Like authority and influence, power aims at compliance, but it does not seek consensus or agreement as a condition of that compliance.

Power is always relational. An individual who has power over another person can narrow that person's range of choice and obtain compliance. The power holder does not necessarily force the compliance by physical acts, but may operate in more subtle ways, such as an implicit threat to carry out sanctions. Latent power is frequently as effective as a show of power. Power attaches to people, not to official positions. The formal authority holder, i.e., the person who has the official title, organizational position, and grant of authority, may or may not have power in addition to this formal grant of authority.

An imbalance in superior-subordinate relationships can occur when a non-officeholder has more power than the official officeholder. This can even be seen in family life. For example, when a two-year-old shows signs of an incipient temper tantrum in the middle of the supermarket, church, or the annual family gathering at the in-laws, the power balance clearly is in favor of the child if the tantrum pattern has developed. The child does not have to carry out the explosive behavior; the mere threat of doing so brings about some desired behavior from the parent caught in the situation. In the privacy of the home, however, the parent-child power balance shifts.

Workers have power over line supervisors and managers. A worker with specific technical knowledge can withhold that key information from a manager or can develop a relationship that is personally favorable. The information may not actually be withheld; the mere possibility that the manager cannot rely on an individual is enough to shift the balance, at least temporarily, in favor of the worker. Groups of workers can control a manager when it is well known that the manager is responsible for meeting a deadline or quota; the manager's ability to do this is dependent on the cooperation of the workers. The normal, steady output may be reached routinely, but that extra push needed to go over the quota or to reach a special level of output rests more with the workers than with the manager. Strikes by workers are classic examples of mobilized power, but the power shifts back in favor of management if striking workers are terminated during a strike.

When an individual can supply something that a person values and cannot obtain elsewhere in a regular manner, or when the individual can deprive this person of something valued, then there is a power relationship. This implicit or explicit power relationship may or may not be perceived by one or both parties.

THE CONCEPT OF INFLUENCE

Like power, influence is the capacity to produce effects on others or to obtain compliance, but it differs from power in the manner in which compliance is evoked. Power is coercive; influence is accepted voluntarily. Influence is the capacity to obtain compliance without relying on formal actions, rules, or force. In relationships of influence, not only compliance, but also consensus and agreement are sought; persuasion rather than latent or overt force is the major factor in influence. Influence supplements power, and it is sometimes difficult to distinguish latent power from influence in a situation. Does the individual comply because of a relationship of influence or because of the latent power factor? Together, power and influence supplement formal authority.

THE CONCEPT OF FORMAL AUTHORITY

Authority may be termed legitimate power. It is the right to issue orders, to direct action, and to command or exact compliance. It is the right given to a manager to employ resources, make commitments, and exercise control. By a grant of formal authority, the manager is entitled, empowered, and authorized to act; thus, the manager incurs a responsibility to act. Authority may be expressed by direct command or instruction or, more commonly, by suggestion. Through the authority delegation, coordination is secured in the organization.

The authority mandate is delineated and reinforced in several ways, such as organization charts, job descriptions, procedure manuals, work rules. Although the exercise of authority in many situations tends to be similar to transactions of influence, authority differs from influence in that authority is clearly vested in the formal chain of command. Individuals are given a specific grant of authority as a result of organizational position. Power and influence may be exercised by an individual authority holder, but they may also be exercised by individuals who do not have a specific grant of authority.

Authority is both complemented and supplemented by power on the one hand and influence on the other. It is within the realm of formal authority to exact compliance by the threat of firing a person; however, this may be such a rare occurrence in an organization that such a threat is really an exercise of power more than an exercise of authority. On the other hand, formal aspects of authority may be so well developed that the major transactions remain at the influence level, with the influence based largely on the holding of formal office. The infrequent use of formal authoritative directives to evoke compliance may indicate organizational health. For the remainder of this discussion, no further distinction between power, influence, and authority will be made.

THE IMPORTANCE OF AUTHORITY

When a subordinate refuses to accept the orders of a superior, the superior has several choices, each carrying potentially negative consequences for the attainment of organizational goals. The superior could accept the insubordination, withdraw the order, and seek to find others to carry out the directive. This action would probably further weaken authority, however, because the superior would be perceived as lacking the subtle blend of power and authority to exact compliance on a predictable basis. A chain reaction of insubordination could occur. If other workers are asked to carry out a directive that had been refused by a worker, resentment could build up with negative consequences. If the order is withdrawn completely, the work will not be accomplished.

The manager who decides to enforce compliance may suspend or fire the insubordinate worker. The superior still must find a worker to carry out the directive. If there is a chain reaction of insubordination, it may become impractical to suspend or fire the entire work force. The situation moves from one of authority to one of power. Therefore, managers must identify and widen their bases of authority to help ensure a stable work climate.

SOURCES OF POWER, INFLUENCE, AND AUTHORITY

The manager's organizational relationships flow along the continuum of power, influence, and authority, varying in emphasis at different times and in different situations. In order to understand more fully the dynamics of the power-influence-authority triad, it is useful to examine the sources or bases of authority in formal organizations. The wider the base of authority, the stronger the manager's position; with a wide base of authority, the manager can work in the realm of influence and need not rely only on the formal grant of authority that flows from organizational position.

The sources of formal authority have been studied by several theorists in the disciplines of social psychology, management, and political science. A review of the literature suggests several sources or bases of authority: (a) the acceptance or consent theories, (b) the theory of formal organizational authority, (c) cultural expectations, (d) technical competence and expertise, and (e) characteristics of the authority holder. The limits or weaknesses of each theory are offset by the approach taken in another.

Acceptance or Consent Theories

The concept that authority involves a subordinate's acceptance of a superior's decision is the basis for the acceptance or consent theory of formal authority. A superior has authority only insofar as the subordinate accepts it. This theory implies that members of the organization have a choice concerning compliance, when often they do not. It remains important to recognize the concepts of acceptance and consent in order to identify the centers of more subtle and diffuse resistance to authority, even when there is no overt and massive insubordination.

The zone of indifference and the zone of acceptance are two similar concepts in the acceptance or consent theory of authority. Chester Barnard[1] used the term *zone of indifference* to describe that area in which an individual accepts orders without conscious questioning. Barnard noted that the manager establishes an overall setting by means of preliminary education, prior persuasive efforts, and known inducements for compliance; the order then lies within the range that is more or less anticipated by the subordinate, who accepts it without conscious questioning or resistance because it is consistent with the overall organizational framework. Herbert Simon used the term *zone of acceptance* to reflect the same authority relationship. The zone of acceptance, according to Simon, is an area established by subordinates within which they are willing to accept the decisions made for them by their superior.[2] Simon noted that this zone is modified by the positive and negative sanctions in the authority relationship, as well as by such factors of community of purpose, habit and leadership.

Coupled with these factors is the concept of the rule of anticipated reactions, which Simon included in his discussion of zone of acceptance.[3] The subordinate seeks to act in a manner that is acceptable to the superior, even when there has been no explicit command. The authority system, including anticipated review of actions, is so well developed that the superior needs only to review actions rather than to issue commands. The past organizational history in which positive and negative sanctions were enforced is recalled; the expectation of the review of actions is fostered so that the subordinate's zone of acceptance is expanded.

Another approach to the concept of authority as a relationship between organizational leaders and their followers is described by Robert Presthus, who posited a transactional view of authority in which there is a reciprocity among individuals at different levels in the hierarchy.[4] Compliance with authority is in some way rewarding to the individual, and this individual, therefore, plays an active role in defining and accepting authority. Everyone has formal authority in that each has a formal role in the organization. There is, Presthus stated, an implicit bargaining and exchange of authority, each deferring to the other.

The notion of reciprocal expectations in authority relationships is further supported in Edgar Schein's discussion of the psychological contract.[5] As it is in Barnard's concept of the zone of indifference and in Simon's rule of anticipated reactions, the premise of member acceptance of organizational authority and its attendant control system is basic to the psychological contract. The worker's acceptance of authority constitutes a realm of upward influence; in turn, the worker expects the authority holders to honor the implicit restrictions on their grant of authority. The worker expects the authority holders to refrain from ordering actions that are inconsistent with the general climate of the given organization and from taking advantage of the worker's acceptance of authority. The worker also expects as part of this psychological contract the rewards of compliance, i.e., positive sanctions readily given and negative sanctions kept at a minimum.

The Theory of Formal Organizational Authority

In his classic study of bureaucracies, Max Weber discussed three forms of authority: charismatic, traditional, and rational-legal. Charisma, as defined by Weber, is a "certain quality of an individual personality by virtue of which he is set apart from ordinary men and treated as endowed with supernatural, superhuman, or at least specifically exceptional qualities."[6] The social, religious, or political groups that form around a charismatic leader tend to lack formal role structure. The routines of bureaucratic structure are not developed and may even be disdained by the group. Charismatic authority figures function as revolutionary forces against established systems of leadership and authority. Charismatic authority is not bound by explicit rules; the authority remains invested in the key charismatic individual. Personal devotion to and an almost irrational faith in the leader bind the members of the group to each other and to the leader.

Since charismatic authority is linked to the individual leader, the organization's survival is similarly linked. If the organization is to endure, it must take on some of the characteristics of formal organizations, including a formalized authority pattern. In this area, two developments are possible. The charismatic leadership may evolve into a traditional system of authority, or it may develop into the rational-legal system of formal authority. In traditionalism, a pattern of succession is developed. A successor may be designated by the leader or hereditary/kinship succession may be established; then a system of transferring the leadership to the legitimate designated individual or heir must be developed. This, in turn, leads to a system of roles and formal authority. Weber uses the term *routinization of charisma* to describe this transformation of charismatic authority into traditional and then into rational-legal authority.

Rational-legal authority is the authority predicated in formal organizations. It is generally assumed that formal organizations come into being and derive legitimacy from an overall social and legal system. Individuals accept authority within the formal organizational structure because the rights and duties of members of the organization are consistent with the more abstract rules that individuals in the larger society accept as legitimate and rational.

Within the formal organization, a system of roles and authority relationships is carefully constructed to enable the organization to survive and move toward its formal goal on a continuing, stable basis. Authority has its basis in the organizational position, not in any individual. Weber described in detail the major characteristics of bureaucratic structures; the following characteristics relate to the rational-legal authority structure:[7]

1. There is the principle of fixed and official jurisdictional areas, which are generally ordered by rules, that is, by laws or administrative regulations.
   a. The regular activities required for the purposes of the bureaucratically governed structure are distributed in a fixed way as official duties.
   b. The authority to give the commands required for the discharge of these duties is distributed in a stable way and is strictly delimited in a fixed way as official duties.

c. Methodical provision is made for the regular and continuous fulfillment of these duties and for the execution of the corresponding rights; only persons who have generally regulated qualifications to serve are employed.

2. The principles of office hierarchy and of levels of graded authority mean a firmly ordered system of superiority and subordination in which there is supervision of the lower offices by the higher ones.

The theory of formal organizational authority rests on this rational-legal system of formal office, impersonality of the officeholder, and a system of rules and regulations to constrain the grant of authority. Delegation of formal authority from top management to each successive level of management is the basis for formal organizational authority. Authority is derived from official position and is circumscribed by the limits imposed by the hierarchical order.

Cultural Expectations

Both the acceptance theory of authority and the formal organizational authority theory include an implicit assumption that individuals in a society are culturally induced to accept authority. Furthermore, the acceptable use of authority in organizations is defined in part by the larger societal mores, as well as by union contract, corporate law, and state and federal law and regulation.

Acceptance of the status system in a society is learned as part of the general socialization process. General deference to authority is ingrained early in the psychosocial development of the child, and social roles with their sanctions are accepted and reinforced throughout adult life. The role of employee carries with it both formal and informal sanctions; insubordination is not generally condoned. Even as a group cheers the occasional rebel, there is an attendant discomfort because something is out of order in the relationship. When the insubordination of an individual begins to threaten the economic security of the group, there is counterpressure on that individual to bring about reacceptance of authority. Fear of authority may bring about a similar response of renewed acceptance of authority and counterpressure on any dissidents.

The expected zone of acceptance or zone of indifference varies with different social roles. These variables are rarely spelled out in great detail; they are learned as much through the pervasive cultural formation process as through the formal orientation process in any one organization. There is a kind of group mind that includes the general realization that a particular behavior pattern is part of a given role, and the entire role set reinforces this general acceptance of authority.

Technical Competence and Expertise

Three terms reflect the organizational authority that is derived from or based on the technical competence and expertise of the individual, regardless of what office or position the individual holds in the organization. These terms are *functional authority, the law of the situation,* and *the authority of facts.*

Functional authority is the limited right that line or staff members (or departments) may exercise over specified activities for which they are responsible (see Line and Staff Relationships, Chapter 5). Functional authority is given to the line or staff member as an exception to the principle of unity of command. For the purposes of this discussion on the sources of authority, it is useful to emphasize the special character of functional authority: It is given to a line or staff member primarily because that individual has specialized knowledge and technical competence. For example, the personnel manager normally assists all other department heads in matters of employee relations, although this manager has no authority to intervene directly in manager-employee relations. The situation changes when there is a legally binding collective bargaining agreement; the personnel manager, with special training in labor relations, may be given functional authority over all matters stemming from the union contract because of specialized knowledge. Another example is that of data processing staff who, because of technical competence, are given authority to make final decisions over certain aspects of data collection. The authority is granted because of the technical competence of the individual.

Mary Parker Follett, a pioneer in management thought, introduced the terms *the law of the situation* and *authority of facts.*[8] Follett described the ideal authority relationship as that stemming from the situation as a whole. Each participant in the organization, who is assumed to have the necessary qualifications for the position held, has authority tied to position. Orders become depersonalized in that each participant in the process studies and accepts the factors in the situation as a whole. Follett stated that one *person* should not give orders to another *person,* but that both should agree to take their orders from the situation.[9] She developed this concept further; both the employer and the employee should study the situation and should apply their specialized knowledge and technical competence through the principles of scientific management. The emphasis shifts, in Follett's approach, from authority derived from official position or office to authority derived from the situation. The individual who has the most knowledge and competence to make the decision and issue the order in a particular situation has the authority to do so. The staff assistant or a key employee has as much authority in a particular situation as does a holder of hierarchical office.

Closely tied to the concept of the law of the situation is that of authority of facts. Follett stressed that, in modern organizations, individuals exercise authority and leadership because of their expert knowledge.[10] Again, the leadership and authority shift from the hierarchical position to the situation. The one with the knowledge demanded by the situation tends to exercise effective authority.

In both of these concepts, there is an emphasis on the depersonalization of orders. At the same time, the source of the authority is highly personal in that knowledge and competence for the exercise of authority is in an individual. Underlying the concepts of functional authority, law of the situation, and authority of facts is the theme that authority is derived from the technical competence and knowledge of individuals in the organization who do not necessarily hold formal office in the line hierarchy.

Characteristics of Authority Holder

Authority rests in individuals. The talents and traits of the individual may become the source of authority, as they do for the charismatic leader. A person holding power may use this as a base for gaining legitimate authority; a group may invest the person of power with legitimate authority as a protective measure and seek to impose the limits and customs of authority. They may also accept the power holder as formal officeholder as a means of accepting the situation without further conflict. Technical competence and knowledge are also personal characteristics that become the basis of authority in certain situations.

The Manager's Use of Authority Sources

In practice, managers should recognize all the potential sources of authority and should weigh the contribution of each theory to obtain as complete a picture of the authority nexus as possible. They should assess their own grant of authority and try to determine which elements tend to strengthen their authority and which tend to erode it.

The base of authority shifts from time to time. For example, an individual is offered the position of department head of the medical record service because of that individual's competence in the administration of medical record systems; this specialized knowledge and technical competence is the first pillar of authority. When the individual accepts the position, the formal authority mandate of that official position is added. This authority, in turn, is shaped by the prevailing organizational climate, which includes a wide or narrow zone of acceptance on the part of employees. The personal traits of the authority holder complete the authority base for that office.

The individual with a participative management style may emphasize those aspects of authority that widen the zone of acceptance. The setting itself may dictate the predominant authority base, as in the law of the situation; in a highly technical setting, those with the most technical knowledge use this knowledge as the base of authority. Although there is a tendency to downplay internal politics in organizations such as health care institutions, some individual managers may use power as a major source of authority. Astute managers regularly assess the several bases of authority available to them in order to enhance the authority relationships and thereby contribute more effectively to the achievement of organizational goals.

RESTRICTIONS ON THE USE OF AUTHORITY

Several factors restrict the use of authority. Some constraints stem from internal factors, such as the limits placed on authority at each organizational level; others stem from external factors such as laws, regulations, and ethical considerations. The following is a systematic summary of these factors:

1. organizational position. Each holder of authority receives a limited delegation of authority consistent with the position held in the organization. An individual has no legitimate formal authority beyond that accorded to the organizational position.
2. legal and contractual mandates. Authority is limited by the federal, state, and municipal laws and regulations relating to safety, work hours, licensure, and scope of practice; by internal corporate charter and bylaws; and by union contract.
3. social limitations. The social codes, mores, and values of the overall society include both implicit and explicit limits on the behavior of individuals. Authority holders are expected to act in a manner consistent with the predominant value system of the society. These social limitations are major factors in shaping the zone of acceptance and the general cultural deference of individuals who are members of organizations.
4. physical limits. An authority holder cannot force a person to do something that is simply beyond that person's physical capabilities, nor can an authority holder escape the natural limits of the physical environment, such as climate or physical laws.

5. technological constraints. The advances and the limitations of the state of the art must be considered in the exercise of authority; no amount of power or authority can bring about a result that is beyond the technical ability of the individuals.
6. economic constraints. The availability of scarce resources limits the behavior of formal authority holders.
7. zone of acceptance of organization members. Both authority and power have their limits in that the net cost of using either must be calculated. When a weak manager is faced with a strong employee group, as in a strong union setting, the cost of using even legitimate authority may be too high; the authority grant is actually diminished.

Although many employees do not have complete freedom to choose what they will or will not do, they may resist authority in subtle ways, such as adherence to job duties exactly as stated in the job description, passive resistance, and failure to take initiative in any area not specifically designated by the supervisor. The manager must move into a distinct leadership position to develop a wide zone of acceptance, as leadership becomes an essential adjunct to the exercise of authority.

LEADERSHIP

The leader goes before and/or with the group to show the way; the leader guides, directs, and influences the group, who more or less willingly accept this influence. Leadership is tied to the need for action. Leadership is the influencing of individuals to strive willingly toward the objectives of the group; it is the art of inducing members to accept and accomplish the work necessary to reach the objective. Leadership is distinguished from power in that force is not a factor in leadership as it is in power relationships. Leadership is also distinct from authority, which is a formal relationship of administrative control. In its pure form, leadership always implies free choice to follow.

Leadership exists both informally and formally. Informal leadership is exerted in many settings, including formal organizations. Within any formal organization, there are subunits and even paraorganizations, such as a collective bargaining unit, that are led by individuals who do not hold formal hierarchical office. Leadership is implied, even explicitly included, in the role of the manager whose function is to achieve organizational objectives by coordinating, motivating, and directing the work group. For the remainder of this discussion on formal leadership, the presumption is made that the manager is a leader in addition to being a holder of formal authority. Philip

Selznick stressed leadership as an attribute of the manager, pointing out that leadership is needed to make critical decisions. The institutional leader is the unique possessor of systems perspective, and this quality, Selznick noted, distinguishes a leader from the individual who is adept in interpersonal relationships.[11]

The Qualities of a Leader

In order to influence and induce others to strive toward a goal, the leader must possess not only a deep vision of that goal, but also the ability to render the goal meaningful to the group. The knowledge, insight, and skill of the leader are greater than those of other members of the group. At an obvious level, the leader leads but does not drag, coerce, or push the group; the group members are steadily induced to move toward the goal. They are influenced in a pervasive way so that the overall goal becomes their own goal. The leader does not achieve the work alone, but rather successfully coordinates the work of the group. The leader inspires confidence through both emotional and knowledge ties with the followers.

The Functions of the Leader

In formal organizations, the leader has certain functions that are tied to the organizational need for leadership. The leader is expected to influence, persuade, and control the group. As the individual with vision, the leader is expected to take calculated risks and to be a catalytic agent in the change process.

The leader carries out important functions on behalf of group members through the role of representative; for example, employees look to their unit or department head to speak for them and to seek to obtain advantages for them. The leader may be cast in several roles by followers, especially at the symbolic level, and may even be seen as the father figure who shields the individual from difficulties. The leader may also be the scapegoat; as the management representative closest to the rank and file worker, the leader/manager bears the brunt of anger when the organizational situation is less than optimal.

The leader is presumed to embody the values of the group. As such, the leader becomes the focal point in the motivational process. Warren Bennis summarized the functions of the leader in his statements concerning an "agricultural" model of leadership. Bennis offered as the major function of the leader the development of the climate and conditions that favor individual involvement in group effort. Leadership is a process more than a structure;

the leader creates the climate for change so that the organization will have the adaptability needed for its survival.[12]

Styles of Leadership

The manner in which a manager interacts with subordinates reflects a cluster of characteristics that constitute a style of leadership. While any manager uses several styles of leadership, choosing the one most appropriate for a given situation, one style generally emerges as that manager's predominant mode of interaction.

Autocratic Leadership

Also referred to as authoritarian, boss-centered, or dictatorial, autocratic leadership is characterized by close supervision. The manager who employs this technique gives direct, clear, and precise directions to employees, telling them what is to be done and how it will be done; there is no room for employee initiative. Employees do not participate in the decision-making process. There is a high degree of centralization and a narrow span of management. The chain of command is clearly and fully understood by all. Autocratic managers use their authority as their principal, or only, method of getting work done because they feel that employees could not properly or efficiently carry out work assignments without detailed instruction.

Although this style of leadership apparently gets results, it can be fatal over the long run. Employees easily lose interest in their assignments and stop thinking for themselves, since there is no occasion for independent thought. Under certain conditions and with specific employees, however, a degree of close supervision may be necessary. Some employees prefer to receive clear and precise orders, because close supervision reassures them that they are doing a good job. Even so, it can generally be assumed that the autocratic, close leadership style is the least effective and least desirable method for motivating employees to optimum performance.

Bureaucratic Leadership

Like the autocratic leader, the bureaucratic leader tells employees what to do and how to do it. The basis for this leadership style is almost exclusively the institution's rules and regulations. For the bureaucrat, these rules are the laws. The bureaucratic manager is normally afraid to take chances and manages "by the book." Rules are strictly enforced, and no departure or exceptions are permitted. The bureaucrat, like the autocrat, permits employees little or no freedom.

Participative Leadership

In participative leadership, the contribution of the group to the organizational effort is emphasized. This style is the opposite of autocratic, close supervision. The manager who employs the participative method involves the employees in the decision-making process and in the maintenance of cohesive group interaction. The manager consults with employees concerning goals and objectives, work assignments, and the extent and content of a problem before making a final decision and issuing directives or orders. This approach is an attempt to make full use of the talents and abilities of the group members; the manager is the facilitator of this process. It is difficult for employees who have participated in the consultative process not to accept the resulting decision.

Some managers use a pseudoparticipative method of leadership to give employees the feeling that consultation has taken place. Employees quickly sense that the manager is manipulating people, however, and that their participation in the decision-making process is not real. The manager who employs the participative style of leadership must take it seriously and must be willing to listen to and evaluate employees' opinions and suggestions before making a final decision.

Participative management does not weaken a manager's formal authority, since the manager retains the right to make the final decision. The obvious advantage of the participative style of leadership revolves around the meaningful involvement of the employees, which greatly enhances the implementation of the decisions that have been made.

Laissez-faire Leadership

Laissez-faire or "free rein" leadership is based on the assumption that individuals are self-motivated. Employees receive little or no supervision. Employees, as individuals or as a group, determine their own goals and make their own decisions. The manager, whose contribution is minimal, acts primarily as a consultant and does so only when asked. The manager does not lead, but allows the employees to lead themselves. Some managers consider this approach true democratic leadership, but the usual end result is disorganization and chaos. The lack of leadership permits different employees to proceed in different directions.

Paternalistic Leadership

The manager who is paternalistic treats employees like children. The manager tells employees what is to be done, but does so in a nice way. It is the paternalistic manager's belief that employees do not really know what is good for them or how to make decisions for themselves. In this approach, everyone is watched over by the benevolent manager—the benign dictator—and the employees eventually become extremely dependent on their "paternalistic boss."

Continuum of Leadership Styles

Another way to view leadership behavior is on a continuum, ranging from highly boss-centered to highly group-centered.[13] The relationship between the manager and the employee in the continuum ranges from completely autocratic, in which there is no employee participation in the decision-making process, to completely democratic, in which the employee participates in all phases of the decision-making process (Figure 8–1). The following is a brief description of the seven gradations along the continuum:

Figure 8-1 Continuum of Leadership Behavior

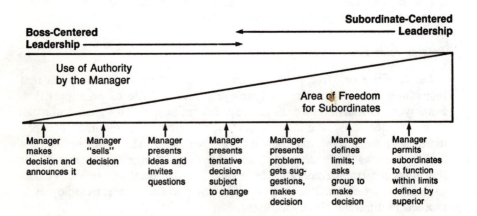

1. *Manager makes decision and announces it.* The manager identifies a problem, considers alternative solutions, selects a course of action, and tells employees what they are to do. Employees do not participate in the decision-making process.
2. *Manager "sells" decision.* The manager again makes the decision without consulting the employees. Instead of announcing the decision, however, the manager attempts to persuade the employees to accept it. The manager details how the decision fits both the goals of the department and the interests of group members.
3. *Manager presents ideas and invites questions.* The manager has made the decision, but asks the employees to express their ideas. Thus, the manager allows for the possibility that the initial decision may be modified.
4. *Manager presents tentative decision subject to change.* The manager allows the employees the opportunity to exert some influence before the decision is finalized. The manager meets with the employees and presents the problem and a tentative decision. Before the decision is finalized, the manager obtains the reactions of employees who will be affected by it.
5. *Manager presents problem, gets suggestions, makes decision.* Up to this point on the continuum, the manager has always come before the employees with at least a tentative solution to the problem. At this point, however, the employees get the first opportunity to suggest solutions. Consultation with the employees increases the number of possible solutions to the problem. The manager then selects the solution that he or she regards as most appropriate in solving the problem.
6. *Manager defines limits; asks group to make decision.* For the first time, the employees make the decision. The manager now becomes a member of the group. Before doing this, however, the manager defines the problem and the limits and boundaries within which the decision must be made.
7. *Manager permits subordinates to function within limits defined by superior.* For the maximum degree of employee participation, the manager defines the problem and lists the guidelines and boundaries within which a solution must be achieved. The limitation imposed on the employees comes directly from the manager, who participates as a group member in the decision-making process and is committed in advance to implementing whatever decision the employees make.

In summary, the manager's relationship with the employees influences morale, job satisfaction, and work output. Employee satisfaction is positively associated with the degree to which employees are permitted to participate in the decision-making process. On the other hand, poor supervision causes employee dissatisfaction, high turnover rates, and low morale.

Factors That Influence Leadership Style

No one style of leadership fits all situations. A successful manager selects a method appropriate for a given situation. Before selecting a style of leadership or deciding to blend several styles, the manager must consider a number of factors:

1. work assignment. If the work assignment is repetitious, the properly trained employee does not need constant or close supervision. If the assignment is new or complex, however, close supervision may be required.
2. personality and ability of the employee. Employees who are not self-starters react best to close supervision. Others, by reason of their personality and work background, can take on new and important responsibilities on their own; these individuals react best to participative leadership. The occupational makeup of a department may also influence the leadership style used by the manager. For professional people (e.g., physical therapists, occupational therapists, medical records personnel) or other highly skilled employees, the employee-centered participative leadership style is often most effective. When employees are unskilled or unable to act independently, the boss-centered or autocratic style of leadership may produce better results.
3. attitude of employee toward the manager. Managers cannot begin to lead or influence behavior unless they are accepted by the group. Employees give managers their authority only when they believe that the goals and objectives of the managers are consistent with their own personal and professional interests.
4. personality and ability of the manager. The manager's personality has a very definite effect on the behavior and performance of employees. The manager must treat employees' opinions and suggestions with respect and must sincerely encourage employee participation.

When faced with different work group encounters and situational factors, the good manager shifts from one style of leadership to another, often without conscious recognition of a shift in style. Table 8–1 shows examples of the adjustments in leadership style that a manager makes in order to influence and stimulate maximum effort from employees.

Table 8-1 Variables in Leadership Style

Work Group	Key Activities or Situation	Leadership Style
Hospital transporters	Transport of patients Safety considerations Schedule considerations Mode of transport	Bureaucratic—policies and procedures must be followed.
Staff physical therapist with experience	Patient evaluation "Need evaluation today." Neurological case Conference at 10:00 A.M.	Laissez-faire—manager does not need to tell physical therapist such typical evaluation elements as motor, sensory, and cognitive tests.
Total physical therapy professional staff (5 physical therapists)	Vacation schedules Consideration of patients, students, and overall coverage One staff resignation in July	Participative—manager consults with employees concerning vacation schedule and the need for proper coverage during the summer months.
Staff physical therapist	Call from physician to staff therapist. Wishes to see therapist at patient's bedside promptly at 9:15 or "Sorry to interrupt but just had a call from Dr. Jones and he requests you be at the patient's room, #343 in 5 minutes."	Autocratic, Nonnegotiable. *Note:* Even, nice tone.

ORDERS AND DIRECTIVES

The manager's role is to direct the employees toward achieving the goals and objectives of the department and the institution. Regardless of the leadership style employed, the manager must issue orders and directives to indicate what must be done. The terms *orders* and *directives* may be used interchangeably, although *orders* has a more autocratic tone.

Giving orders is a major function of the manager's day-to-day operation of the program. Too often, it is taken for granted that every manager knows how to give orders. Unfortunately, this is not always true. The manager must remember to convey to the employees *what* is to be done, *who* is to do it, and *when, where, how,* and *why.* At times, some of the components are implied or omitted. For example, "Effective July 1, John Doe will be the Senior Physical Therapist of the Amputee Service." This statement answers the *what, who, when,* and *where,* but omits the *how* and *why.*

Verbal Orders vs. Written Orders

The form of an order depends on the situation. The verbal order is the most frequently used. Because it is given on a one-to-one basis with immediate feedback, the manager can observe the employee's reaction, ask questions, and appraise the degree of understanding. Disagreements can be handled immediately. Observation of the employee's body language provides additional feedback.

When permanence is important, written orders are more appropriate. This form is most effective when information is to be disseminated to employees as a group. Written orders are more carefully thought through, since there is less opportunity for explanation. The use of long sentences, excessive adjectives, and involved word patterns should be avoided. The written order also carries a degree of formality not present in the verbal order. It is difficult, however, to keep written material up-to-date and impossible to clear up obscure meanings.

Making Orders Acceptable and Effective

The issuing of effective orders requires attention to timing and language. Planning to issue the order involves content, format (oral or written), and the manner in which the order is actually issued. When there is rapport between the manager and employee, a simple request may be suitable; an implied order is sometimes given with the same informality. When certain action must be taken, precision is involved, or misunderstanding must be avoided, the written, direct order is the best method. The sense of command may be foreign to many managers, yet commands may be needed on some occasions, such as emergencies. Although policies, work rules, and procedures may not be considered orders, they fall into the category of the required course of action as determined by management.

Since a critical aspect of the manager's function is communicating, effort must be given to making orders acceptable and effective. Acceptability is enhanced by the general processes of leadership that the manager has developed over time. In effect, the manager prepares the employees in many ways so that, when orders are actually given, they are normally both acceptable and effective in terms of essential communication.

DISCIPLINE

The attitudes and emotions of each employee within an organization not only affect the degree to which goals and objectives are met, but also influence the behavior of all employees within a group setting. The manager of any unit or department must be concerned with the conduct or discipline of all employees within that unit or department. This can best be accomplished by establishing reasonable standards of conduct or work rules, informing employees of these standards, and enforcing them wisely.

Because the word *discipline* is immediately associated with the use of authority, it carries the disagreeable connotation of punishment. Discipline should be used to improve employee behavior, however, and to motivate employees so that they will be self-disciplined and effective in the performance of their jobs. A manager's actions that call attention to correct behavior are more effective in promoting self-discipline and cooperation than those that call attention to incorrect behavior.

Even in an organization where employees have a high degree of self-discipline, a manager must occasionally take some type of disciplinary action because rules have been broken. At this point, the manager is confronted with a situation in which the more restricted meaning of discipline is required. Disciplining becomes a response to unacceptable behavior, and the imposition of penalties is the only course open to the manager for correcting the employee's behavior and maintaining control of the department. Distasteful as it may be, it is the manager's responsibility to act promptly, firmly, and consistently. This means that disciplinary action should follow the misconduct as closely as possible. Since harsh words may be exchanged during the discussion, the manager must maintain self-control. The manager who feels that loss of control is a risk should avoid taking any action until a later date.

The manager must handle all disciplinary action as a private matter. If the manager can be overheard in disciplining, the other employees of the department will judge the manager's performance. Being observed or overheard by others may only confuse the situation and foster ill feelings among the manager, the employee, and co-workers. This situation may further damage manager-employee relationships. Therefore, privacy during any disciplinary action is essential.

Progressive Disciplinary Action

When an institution has a union contract, the disciplinary process is usually outlined in the policy and procedure manual or in the work rules of the institution. Many institutions that do not have these documents have accepted the idea of progressive discipline, which has become fairly well standardized as a result of custom and practice. In order of increasing severity, these are as follows:

1. general counseling
2. oral warning with a notation in the employee's employment record
3. official written warning noted in the employment record
4. disciplinary layoff without pay, varying in length from one day to two weeks
5. termination

Consistent with the concept of positive, corrective discipline, oral or written warnings are given for minor offenses. The oral warning is used when it is believed that the employee does not fully understand the significance of the actions or behavior. It is hoped that emphasizing the need for a change in behavior at this point will make further disciplinary action unnecessary. The employee who continues to violate established standards should be warned in writing. The warning should state how the employee's performance or conduct is unacceptable and what particular punishment is prescribed by institutional rules and regulations for continued infractions. A copy of the warning should be given to the employee and a duplicate copy placed in the employee's personnel file so that it becomes a part of the employee's permanent record (Exhibit 8–1).

The disciplinary layoff may be used when all previous disciplinary steps have produced no change in the employee's behavior. The length of the disciplinary layoff depends on the seriousness of the offense and the number of times it has been repeated; it may vary from one day to several weeks. An employee who continues misconduct after oral warnings and an official written warning will find a disciplinary layoff without pay a rude awakening.

Termination is the most severe form of disciplinary action and should be used only for the most serious offenses, such as stealing, falsification of records, drinking of alcoholic beverages, or use of narcotics during work time, or for a record of repeated offenses. When termination is necessary, every effort should be made by management to maintain pleasant relationships with the employee who is about to be terminated.

In all disciplinary actions, the time element is important. How long should an infraction of the rules and regulations of the institution be held against an employee? Current practice is to wipe the slate clean and disregard offenses committed one or two years ago. There is no justification for continual reference to offenses of past years if the employee has maintained a good record for at least one year.

Exhibit 8–1 Official Written Warning

May 18
To: S. Jennings
From: H. Morgan, Director of Physical Therapy
Subject: Lateness

On February 22, I counseled you regarding your frequent lateness and cautioned you about the continued violation of this specific work rule. I also reviewed that portion of the work rules, Section 5, Lateness, for the exact wording and the need to conform to established procedures. On two separate occasions after this, we again discussed your pattern of late arrival. Verbal warnings were issued on March 15 and April 3.

Since February 22, your pattern of late arrival has continued. Therefore, on this date, May 18, in my office, we again discussed your failure to be at work at the designated time of 8:30 A.M. This memorandum is to confirm our conversation and to issue an official written warning that continuation of frequent lateness could result in progressive disciplinary action as noted in the work rules of the institution.

A copy of this memorandum has been placed in your personnel file.

The disciplinary action used by the manager should match the severity of the offense, and the manager must remember that the purpose of the action is to correct the employee's behavior and to avoid similar offenses in the future. Whatever disciplinary action is taken, it should be done on an impersonal basis. It is the specific offense that requires discipline, not the personality of the employee. If the manager criticizes the offense, not the employee, the individual is likely to accept discipline more willingly.

Appeal Procedure

In every organization, there must be a grievance procedure whereby employees have the right to appeal a disciplinary action that they feel is unfair. If an employee belongs to a union, the right of appeal and the grievance procedure is specifically outlined in the union-management contract. (A typical grievance process under a union contract is included in Chapter 15.) The right of appeal should also be available to an employee of an institution where there is not a union. In either situation, the grievance procedure is an orderly way of resolving conflict. In most cases, the appeal process follows the chain of command. The privilege of appealing disciplinary action through a specified grievance procedure gives the employees confidence in being treated fairly.

TRAINING

A basic responsibility of every manager is to shape and modify the behavior of employees so that they have the necessary knowledge, skill, and attitude to perform their assignments according to the policies, rules, and regulations of the institution. Advances in technology necessitate continual retraining of experienced employees to perform new and changed tasks. Training and staff development become the fundamental approach by which behavior can be changed in order to meet both the immediate and long-range needs of the institution.

An organized formal training program to meet certain objectives is the most effective method of changing the behavior of employees. To establish such a program, the manager and those individuals involved in the organized training program must (1) identify the training needs, (2) establish training objectives, (3) select appropriate methods and techniques, (4) implement the program, and (5) evaluate the training outcomes.

Identification of Training Needs

The need for training must be specified before the program can be instituted. Training needs are identified through job analyses and job descriptions; they can be classified in two basic categories: (1) immediate needs and (2) future needs. Both the immediate and long-range training needs must be considered if the program is to contribute to the goals and objectives of the organization.

Training Objectives

Once training needs have been identified, the objectives for the program must be established. The objectives should be written in measurable terms and should state the specific outcomes to be achieved at the conclusion of the training program. For example, if a training program for physical therapists is to introduce the Subjective, Objective, Assessment, Plan (SOAP) for writing notes, the manager must establish an objective that states, "Record physical therapy progress notes using the SOAP format for all patients receiving treatment in the department." This objective is specific and stated in measurable terms, since the desired results can be factually determined through record keeping. Written objectives serve as the fundamental guide for organizing the program and evaluating the desired outcomes.

Training Methods and Techniques

The manager has many training methods available to achieve the desired outcomes. The methods most often used are

- job rotation. This technique is a popular approach to staff training and development. Under a rotational schedule, job assignments usually last anywhere from three to six months. This approach gives an employee the opportunity to acquire the broad perspective and diversified skills needed for professional and personal development. Job rotation can also be used to introduce new concepts and ideas into the various units within the department and to help individual employees to think in terms of the whole program rather than their immediate assignments.

- formal lecture presentations. The lecture method is one of the oldest techniques used in training and development programs. The fundamental purpose of the lecture is to inform. The lecture format saves time because the speaker can present more material in a given amount of time than can be presented by any other method. The lecture should be supplemented by visual aids, however, or the results are likely to fall short of the instructional goals. During the lecture, employees are passive. Outside disturbances or mental wanderings frequently distract individuals and, therefore, render the lecture ineffective.

- seminars and conferences. The major purpose of seminars and conferences is to allow for the exchange of ideas, discussion of problems, finding answers to questions or solutions to problems. The opportunity for employees to express their own views and to hear other opinions can be very stimulating. Employees who actively participate are more committed to decisions than they would be if the solution were merely presented to them. It must be remembered that learning takes place in direct ratio to the amount of individual involvement in the discussion process.

- role playing. Acting out situations between two or more persons is a training method used successfully with all levels of employees. Interviewing, counseling, leadership, and human relations are a few of the content areas in which role playing has been used. By playing the role of others, employees gain valuable insight not only from their own action, but from the comments of observers.

- committee assignments. Through committee assignments, employees can explore a topic or problem to gain a wider or new perspective, experience situations involving the resolution of different ideas, learn to adjust to someone else's viewpoint, and practice reaching decisions. Committee assignments also offer opportunities for employees to assume positions of leadership that they would not otherwise have.

- case study. Based on the premise that solving problems under simulated conditions enables employees to solve similar problems in an actual work situation, the case study method requires the employees or a group to become actively involved in a problem-solving situation, either hypothetical or real. The case studies used in developing problem-solving skills should be carefully selected and pertinent to the job so that their use meets the training and development requirements of the employees.

Program Implementation

Throughout the implementation phase, the physical and psychological environment must be constantly monitored. For example, the time schedule, the learning environment, and the pace need to be checked periodically.

The primary consideration in any training program is to establish a time schedule to provide the greatest educational impact possible without reducing work output or, in health care institutions, patient care. The training program and the methods to be used should be announced well in advance. This allows everyone involved sufficient lead time to arrange individual schedules so that work assignments can be adequately covered during the employee's absence.

The arrangement of the room can either promote or handicap the process of learning. It is important to ensure that each participant see and hear each member of the group. The traditional classroom setting in which the "teacher" sits in the front of the room and the participants are seated in neat rows should be avoided whenever possible because it creates a stiff and formal atmosphere. One of the best approaches for a training session is to arrange the tables in an open-ended rectangle, with chairs placed only on the outside perimeter. In addition to the physical arrangement, the room should be well lighted and adequately ventilated.

The pace and timing of each session are also important during the implementation phase of a training program. The function of pace is to maintain interest; therefore, the pace should be quickened when interest begins to sag, or it should be slowed if individuals are having difficulty absorbing content. A training session should not last longer than two hours if learning is to be maximal. In fact, a one-hour session is believed to produce better results. If a two-hour session is necessary, a break should be allowed at the midpoint. Common sense and individual attention spans dictate how long adults accustomed to active work can be kept relatively immobile.

Evaluation of Outcomes

Probably the most difficult aspect of the training program is to evaluate the desired outcomes, because there are no concrete and precise measuring tools to determine changes in behavior and attitudes. Outcomes must be measured indirectly and conclusions based on inference. The evaluation is not just a single act or event, but an entire process. If objectives have been clearly stated in measurable terms, however, evaluation is easier.

A before-after comparison may be a useful way of evaluating change. If the manager and those individuals involved in the training program assess the behavior factors they wish to change before training and examine the same factors after the training has been concluded, they can determine if a change occurred.

Employee training must be undertaken on behalf of and by all employees of a work unit or department. Employee training cannot be done only occasionally. It must be an ongoing activity used when and where it is needed, not just window dressing to impress administration or accreditation agencies.

NOTES

1. Chester Barnard, *The Functions of the Executive* (Cambridge, MA: Harvard University Press, 1968), pp. 167–169.

2. Herbert Simon, *Administrative Behavior* (New York: Macmillan, 1965), p. 12.

3. Ibid., p. 129.

4. Robert Presthus, "Authority in Organizations," in *Concepts and Issues in Administrative Behavior,* eds. Sidney Mailick and Edward H. Van Ness (Englewood Cliffs, NJ: Prentice Hall, 1962), p. 122.

5. Edgar H. Schein, *Organizational Psychology* (Englewood Cliffs, NJ: Prentice Hall, 1965), p. 11.

6. H.H. Gerth and C. Wright Mills, *From Max Weber: Essays in Sociology* (New York: Oxford University Press, 1946), pp. 196–204.

7. Ibid.

8. H.C. Metcalf and L. Urwick, eds., *Dynamic Administration: The Collected Papers of Mary Parker Follett* (New York: Harper, 1942).

9. Ibid.

10. Ibid.

11. Philip Selznick, *Leadership in Administration* (Evanston, IL: Row, Peterson Co., 1957).

12. Warren Bennis, "New Patterns of Leadership," in *Health Care Administration: A Managerial Perspective,* eds. Samuel Levy and N. Paul Loomba (Philadelphia: J.B. Lippincott, 1973), p. 163.

13. Robert Tannenbaum and Warren H. Schmidt, "How to Choose a Leadership Pattern," *Harvard Business Review* 36, no. 2 (1958): 96–101.

Chapter 9

Communication

CHAPTER OBJECTIVES

1. Define the various levels of communication.
2. Develop methods to promote personal communication.
3. Identify behaviors and situations that block communication.
4. Analyze the communication tools used by organizations.
5. Develop a personal communication style that is effective in a variety of communication settings—interpersonal relationships, small and large groups, or organizations.

In a large organization, decisions are usually presented as orders, and members are asked to comply. Work roles are specialized, and communication is carried out by means of formal channels, such as memos, regulations, and lectures. The situation is quite different with a small organization, e.g., one that has less than 20 people. Work roles overlap and are less specialized. Communication is informal, and the opportunity for shared information is increased. Formal communication is minimal. Clearly, just one factor, size, can influence the quality and type of communication used in an organization.

There are many other factors to consider. Communication is a complex process that requires skills on both an individual and group level. As one person interacts with more and more people, the complexity of the interaction also increases.

DEFINITION

Communication is an exchange of ideas, thoughts, or emotions between two or more people. Humans can also communicate with animals, and animals can communicate with each other; however, only humans exchange symbolic information through complex patterns of thought that are transmitted by language, gesture, and movement. Communication has a verbal and nonverbal component, with both conscious and unconscious aspects in each.

PERSONAL AND SMALL GROUP COMMUNICATION

Verbal Communication

The three parts of a verbal exchange are the voice, the content of the message and response, and the method in which information is transmitted. The tone of a speaker's voice can convey emotions. The voice quality, which is a physical characteristic, may also affect the communication process. Accents, intonation, speed of delivery, and use of silence are all part of a verbal exchange.[1]

The unconscious aspects of verbal communication are frequently overlooked. Conscious information is volitional because the speaker is aware of the content, direction, and reasons for the exchange. In greetings, information sharing, confrontations, and discussions, for example, the speaker can identify the reasons for the communication. On the other hand, there may be unconscious motives for the verbal communication, such as thoughts, aspirations, desires, anxieties, fears, or emotions that influence behavior but are hidden from the person's conscious thoughts. A slip of the tongue is an example of an unconscious verbalization.[2]

Nonverbal Communication

Comprised of movements, gestures, expressions, and silences, nonverbal communication may or may not accompany verbal communication. People may not speak, and yet ideas are exchanged. For example, telephone conversations are dependent on the voice, but intonation and silences frequently convey information beyond the spoken words. Two people who share a "knowing" look while waiting for a third have shared an idea without uttering a word.

Nonverbal communication can have both conscious and unconscious aspects. As discussed earlier, conscious information is available for analysis and scrutiny. Unconscious thoughts also influence behavior, but these thoughts, feelings, or emotions are not part of the person's awareness. Analysis of the content of thoughts is difficult because the forces are hidden.

Table 9–1 Examples of Personal Communication

	Verbal	Nonverbal
Conscious	Speeches, greetings	Wave hello, nod head to affirm interest
Unconscious	Slip of the tongue, mistake in verbalizing	Cross legs away from speaker, smirk while hearing suggestion

Communication levels can be presented on a matrix. Table 9–1 is based on the Johari Window which was developed by Joseph Luft and appeared in many group dynamics texts and courses in the last 20 years.[3]

Body language is a series of conscious or unconscious postures that convey information to others. Many studies, both popular and scholarly, have been done to explore this topic. Popularized versions seem to indicate that gestures are universal. Few gestures are, however; most are culturally bound. A nod of the head may mean yes in one society, but it may mean no in another. Birdwhistel made detailed studies of human gestures and analyzed the complexity of body language.[4] Interpretation of human gestures, expressions, silences, and body movement must be cautious. It is best to check perceptions with the other person.

Communication Distance

Hall discussed four levels of distance that are used by humans during communication.[5] His research was based on observations and interviews with middle-class adults from the northeastern seaboard of the United States. These crude observations are merely a first attempt to develop approximate categories. The four distance zones are

1. intimate distances, from 1 to 18 inches. Individuals are involved in lovemaking, wrestling, comforting, or protecting each other. Verbalizations are involuntary or very quiet.[6]
2. personal distances, from 1½ to 4 feet. Individuals can hold or grasp each other. Visual images are still distorted, but they begin to normalize as the person moves to arm's length. Verbalizations are moderate.[7]
3. social distance, from 4 to 12 feet. Individuals are less intimate. Voice level is normal, and conversations can be overheard. Impersonal business is conducted at this distance, but the interaction becomes more formal as the persons involved move to the 12-foot distance.[8]
4. public distance, from 12 to beyond 25 feet. Voice volume is increased, and details about the person are not noticed. Verbalization is formal.[9]

Impression Management

Verbal, nonverbal, and distance management are used to create impressions on others. Another form of nonverbal communication is the type of clothing, accessories, and jewelry worn by the individual.[10] Image management is a studied attempt to present the self in a predetermined fashion in order to guide the reception received from others. Numerous books have recently appeared to guide the reader's quest for the perfect image. Style, color, posture, and body movements are all props that can be manipulated to emphasize selected parts of one's personality. People can read the image and interact accordingly. The reception that a person wearing dungarees receives at an exclusive club is quite different from the reception received by a person wearing designer jeans and accessories that indicate membership at the club. There is one flaw in the creation of an image—an image cannot last forever. People soon learn if their initial impression does not fit the individual. If the image conflicts with the personality, communication may become difficult.

Components of Communication

Communication has four components: initiation, transmission, reception, and feedback. For communication to occur, there must be a sender, someone who begins the interaction. Initiation, which includes the preparation for the interaction, might begin on a nonverbal level and move to a verbal exchange. Transmission is the movement of the communication from one party to another; it depends on verbal and nonverbal sharing methods. Reception is the manner in which the message is received. The receiver's perception shapes the way in which a message is decoded and acted upon. In order to ensure that the sender and the receiver are truly sharing ideas, the receiver offers feedback, which is a verbal or nonverbal signal that acknowledges the message. Common acknowledgements are action, modification, suppression, or nonacceptance of the information.

Personal communication depends on assumptions, perceptions, feelings, past experiences, and present surroundings. Although people frequently talk, communication may prove taxing and difficult. People must transcend personal and cultural barriers that filter their understanding of an exchange.

Methods To Improve Communication

Communication is improved by observing, attending, responding to requests, and checking information. Each of these depends on an objective analysis of an exchange. Observation is the ability to perceive events, objects, and people. Skilled observers are objective and can separate their own inner world from outside reality. Accurate observation is dependent on self-knowledge, because inner reality can make someone "see" things that did not happen. The event is "real" in the mind of the person who really wants to "see" it.

Attending is the ability to hear or see events as they are. During a conversation, instead of planning their next remark, those who are attending direct their energy toward listening or empathizing with the other person. Attending is also called active listening. Responding is the behavior an individual selects to address the needs or requests of the other person. The behavior may be verbal or nonverbal, and the quality of the response shapes the remainder of the communication. If a person asks for the time and receives a pleasant answer, that person may decide to continue the exchange. In contrast, unpleasant replies may inhibit further communication.

Active listening can also help an individual to decode less obvious requests. Sometimes, a sender makes an indirect request, which may be symbolic or may indicate unconscious requestor desires. A perceptive listener should try to "hear" the request and bring the buried topic into the conversation. For example, Allie asked Mary for her pathology notes. Mary responded by saying that she would be glad to duplicate the notes, and she began to rummage in her purse. Allie handed Mary a tissue. Mary seemed grateful and quickly wiped her nose. Allie then handed Mary some money to cover the cost of duplicating the notes. A less perceptive listener may have mistaken Mary's action as a hint for payment or as a rejection of the request. In reality, Mary's nose was running, and she was distracted for a minute while she attended to it.

Communication is also improved by checking information. Listeners can check information by matching their perception of a situation with the sender's intention. In the example given earlier, Allie could have asked Mary if she needed a tissue. Listeners can examine the validity of their perceptions by paraphrasing the sender's message and asking for feedback.

People must be aware of symbols that may be archetypal, cultural, or idiosyncratic.[11] A symbol is any object, pictorial representation, or art that represents something else. Archetypal symbols are shared by humans and extend back in history; for example, a circle means unity throughout the world. Cultural symbols are specific to a subgroup, such as a thumb extended upward means a victory or a good job. Idiosyncratic symbols are specific to an individual or small group. Men who wear one pierced earring share an idiosyncratic symbol that they are "cool." Symbolic meanings contribute to the variety and breadth of communication by forcing listeners to move beyond their personal understanding of gestures, body movements, expressions, and silences.

Personal Tools To Foster Communication

There are six personal tools to promote communication:

1. authenticity, the ability to be true to one's own feelings.
2. acceptance of feelings, which is based on authenticity. People who accept their own feelings can extend this acceptance to the feelings of others.
3. disclosure, the ability to share feelings, both positive and negative, with others. Honest people are able to share information openly.
4. empathy, the ability to project one's own personality onto another person. This promotes understanding.
5. caring, the desire to help others, on an individual and collective level.[12]
6. humor, the ability to identify situations as ludicrous, comic, or happy.[13]

All six tools require the integration of personal needs with goals and actions.

Communication Barriers

Communication can be blocked by internal or external forces. Internal forces, including both conscious and unconscious thoughts, may preclude listening, sharing, and caring so that the meaning of the exchange is confused and misinterpreted. Conscious behaviors that limit communication are facial expressions that are perceived as negative or inappropriate, e.g., smiling when reprimanding a subordinate; body postures that are perceived as rejecting or critical of the person, e.g., folding one's arms over one's chest although expressing a desire to share ideas; verbalizations that interrupt the flow of the exchange, e.g., saying "fabulous!" every time a speaker pauses; interruption or disruption of the speaker's thoughts, e.g., changing topics abruptly, such as interrupting a request for assistance with a comment about football scores.

External forces also impede communication. Distractions, such as noise, motion, and confusion, compromise the quality of an exchange. The context for a communication adds to or subtracts from the interaction. For example, a crowded room with flashing lights and loud music is designed for sensory stimulation, not verbal communication. In this environment, intimate conversations are taxed and labored; communication is limited to nonverbal cueing.

COMMUNICATION IN ORGANIZATIONS

Communication between two people may be difficult, and small group communication may be taxing; however, the task of communicating in a large group may be overwhelming. Bureaucracies emerged at the turn of the century when industrialization promoted the growth of large organizations. The need to develop complex communication patterns became more pressing as organizations added more and more new members. Communication had to keep pace with production. The resulting strategies to increase organizational communication can be divided into two categories: formal and informal.

Formal Communication

An organization is a stratified social system with a hierarchy of roles. The roles are arranged according to the degree of power and status assigned to each, and the assignment is based on the goal-oriented needs of the organization. Formal communication is sanctioned by the organization and is shared along communication channels that are established by the hierarchy of roles. The arrangement of roles determines the direction of the communication.

Formal communication is directional. The four traditional channels of communication are upward, downward, diagonal, and lateral (Exhibit 9–1).

Formal verbal communication in organizations takes place through orderly channels. The exchanges are directional and promote organizational goals, such as a verbal exchange of orders or instructions. Department meetings can also be formal. An aide who wants to register a complaint must pursue a

Exhibit 9–1 Example of Directionality

Four Channels	Examples
1. Upward	● Staff person communicating with supervisor
2. Downward	● Staff therapist giving orders to an aide
3. Diagonal	● Department head of social work conferring with patient registrar in Admissions
4. Lateral	● Nurse sharing night orders with another nurse

series of formal channels; the aide cannot walk into the president's office and discuss the grievance.

Because the size of organizations precludes face-to-face interaction among the majority of group members, they must rely on nonverbal communication, i.e., written and transmitted communication. Common examples include goal statements, policy manuals, directives, procedure manuals, direct mailings to employees, inserts in pay envelopes, organizational bulletins, newsletters, magazines, bulletin boards, posters, and handbooks.

The use of space is another aspect of nonverbal communication. The goals of the organization determine the location and quality of space assigned to group members (who may resist adjustments and reassignments). The way that furniture is arranged, the selection of ornaments, the care given to the space all reflect the values of the group. If an organization has an elaborate waiting room and sloppy offices, it can be inferred that the company is more interested in its public face.

The arrangement of furniture can stimulate or stifle communication. Managers rely on spatial relationships to strengthen their communication. For example, asking for a raise while the manager looks over a desk is more difficult than asking while both parties are seated next to each other.

Informal Communication

Because informal communication is not sanctioned by the social system, it may or may not promote the goals of the organization. Informal communication is not directional; it may circumvent formal channels. Informal communication may be anonymous, and sources cannot be double-checked.

Informal communication, such as small talk and gossip, may not be accurate. Even so, the use of informal communication should not be neglected. Managers and supervisors can use this type of communication to determine the success of formal communication patterns. Rumor and gossip, although inaccurate, may gauge the feelings of group members. Perceptions about events can also be examined. Informal communication is a barometer of the organization, because information can travel at a fast rate of speed. Future events may be foreshadowed by listening to information communicated informally.

Tools To Improve Communication

A number of formal and informal tools can be used to promote communication. Assessment instruments require an analysis of the conscious and unconscious goals of group members. Some can be used to assess individual interaction styles, members' perceptions of each other, perceptions of leadership, roles that members play with each other in the work group, and members' feelings about the organization. Group members complete questionnaires, and the results are compared and discussed. The goals of the members are compared with the goals of the leaders. The results are discussed in nonthreatening ways. Strategies for promoting change can be generated in the group.

Sometimes, group communication becomes so difficult that outside experts, called facilitators, are brought in to resolve the issues. Facilitators are trained in a number of disciplines, including business, psychology, education, and sociology.

Barriers to Communication in Organizations

A number of factors can block communication or distort the goals of organizational exchanges:

1. language. There may be a lack of common meaning among the participants. The use of slang, jargon, or technical language can create problems.
2. unconscious motives. Inner thoughts, ideas, and emotions that are not readily available for examination may cloud a group's ability to perceive or interpret events. A group may share a collective mentality that may not be based on real events. The collective thought has been shaped by emotions.
3. psychological factors. Past experience and ideas impinge on the communication process. Feelings such as mistrust, fear, anger, hostility, or indifference may shape group perceptions.
4. status. Real or perceived differences in rank, socioeconomic status, or prestige may detract from the communication process. People develop preconceived notions about others and act on their preconceptions instead of reality.
5. organizational size. The larger the social system, the greater the number of communication layers. Each layer provides an opportunity for additional distortion.
6. logistical factors. Groups may lack the time, place, or space to communicate clearly. Feedback may be neglected because it is difficult to collect.
7. overstimulation. Members may be bombarded with so many events that they are unable to process any more information. People who are stressed must be managed carefully so that they are not burdened additionally.

8. cultural clashes. One group may misinterpret another's ideas because of a difference in cultural factors, such as age, socioeconomic status, the region of birth, and education level.
9. organizational structure. Communication may be blocked by the structure of the communication channels. One person's role may serve as a bottleneck for open communication. In another instance, roles may overlap, and some groups may not receive the information that they need.
10. phase in life cycle of organization. Communication may be taxed by the organization's developmental stage. The old channels may not have adapted to new situations. Sometimes, organizations rely on one type of communication and ignore other methods.

NOTES

1. Evelyn W. Mayerson, *Putting the Ill at Ease* (Hagerstown, MD: Harper & Row, 1976), pp. 1–36.

2. Sigmund Freud, *A General Introduction to Psychoanalysis,* trans. Joan Riviere (New York: Washington Square Press, 1964), p. 40.

3. Joseph Luft, *Group Process* (Palo Alto, CA: National Press Books, 1963).

4. R.L. Birdwhistel, *Kinesics and Context* (New York: Ballantine Books, 1970).

5. E.T. Hall, *The Hidden Dimension* (Garden City, NY: Anchor Books, 1966), p. 113.

6. Ibid., pp. 116–119.

7. Ibid., pp. 119–120.

8. Ibid., pp. 121–123.

9. Ibid., pp. 123–125.

10. J.T. Molloy, *The Women's Dress for Success Book* (New York: Warner, 1979).

11. A.C. Mosey, *Three Frames of References for Mental Health* (Thorofare, NJ: Charles B. Slack, 1970), p. 52. Taken from J. Mazer, G. Fidler, L. Kovalenko, and K. Overly, *Exploring How a Think Feels* (New York: American Occupational Therapy Association, 1969).

12. Naomi I. Brill, *Working with People* (Philadelphia: J.B. Lippincott, 1973), pp. 31–46.

13. V.M. Robinson, *Humor & The Health Professions* (Thorofare, NJ: Charles B. Slack, 1977).

Chapter 10

Controlling

CHAPTER OBJECTIVES

1. Define the management function of controlling.
2. Relate controlling to planning.
3. Identify the basic control process.
4. Develop specific tools of control: the Gantt chart, the PERT network, the flow chart, the flow process chart, and the work distribution chart.

Controlling is the management function in which performance is measured and corrective action is taken to ensure the accomplishment of organizational goals. It is the policing operation in management, although the manager seeks to create a positive climate so that the process of control is accepted as part of routine activity. Controlling is also a forward-looking process in that the manager seeks to anticipate deviation and prevent it.

The manager initiates the control function during the planning phase, when possible deviation is anticipated and policies are developed to help ensure uniformity of practice. During the organizing phase, a manager may consciously introduce the "deadly parallel" arrangement as a control factor (see Basic Departmentation, Chapter 5). Close supervision and a tight leadership style reflect an aspect of control. Through rewards and positive sanctions, the manager seeks to motivate workers to conform, thus limiting the amount of control that must be imposed. Finally, the manager develops specific control tools, such as inspections, visible control charts, work counts, special reports, and audits.

THE BASIC CONTROL PROCESS

The control process involves three phases that are cyclic: establishing standards, measuring performance, and correcting deviation. In the first step, the specific units of measure that delineate acceptable work are determined. Basic standards may be stated as staff hours allowed per activity, speed and time limits, quantity that must be produced, and number of errors or rejects permitted. The second step in the control process, measuring performance, involves comparing the work, i.e., the goods produced or the service provided, against the standard. Employee evaluation is one aspect of this measurement. In manufacturing, inspection of goods is a routine part of this process; studies of consumer/client satisfaction are key elements when services are involved. Finally, if necessary, remedial action is taken, including retraining employees, repairing equipment, or changing the quality of raw material for manufactured goods.

CHARACTERISTICS OF ADEQUATE CONTROLS

Several features are necessary to ensure the adequacy of control processes and tools:

- timeliness. The control device should reflect deviations from the standard promptly, at an early stage, so there is only a small time lag between detection and the beginning of corrective action.
- economy. If possible, control devices should involve routine, normal processes rather than the special inspection routines at additional cost. The control devices must be worth their cost.
- comprehensiveness. The controls should be directed at the basic phases of the work rather than later levels or steps in the process; for example, a defective part is best inspected and eliminated before it has been assembled with other parts.
- specificity and appropriateness. The control process should reflect the nature of the activity. Proper laboratory inspection methods, for example, differ from the financial audit and machine inspection processes.
- objectivity. The processes should be grounded in fact, and standards should be known and verifiable.
- responsibility. Controls should reflect the authority-responsibility pattern. As far as possible, the worker and the immediate supervisor should be involved in the monitoring and correction process.
- understandability. Control devices, charts, graphs, and reports that are complicated or cumbersome will not be used readily.

Types of Standards

Standards may be of a physical nature, both in terms of quantity and quality, e.g., pounds of laundry that are clean and without stains or the number of charts processed according to the required regulations. Such standards make it easier to develop inspection processes, because such information can be recorded relatively simply on visible control charts, work logs, and similar tools. Standards may also be set in terms of cost; a monetary value is attached to an operation or to the delivery of a service, e.g., the cost per square foot per employee, the cost per patient per visit, or the cost per object in a factory. Occasionally, the standard is expressed somewhat intangibly, such as the success of a volunteer drive, competence or loyalty in an employee, or ability in a trainee. Whenever possible, however, a quantifiable factor should be introduced. For example, behavioral objectives could be developed for each level of trainee functioning.

The Intangible Nature of Service

Health care organizations face a special difficulty in that their primary activities are services, which do not always lend themselves to quantifiable measurements. Furthermore, it is difficult to monitor the delivery of a service because of its dynamic nature. Patient privacy is a major consideration. Another dilemma stems from attempts to delineate services in terms of cost; many services must remain available even if they are not used every day. A highly specialized burn unit must be ready to receive patients even if the patient census has dropped during a given period. An emergency room must have adequate coverage no matter how many patients come for service at a particular time.

TOOLS OF CONTROL

Certain tools of control may be combined with the planning process. Management by objectives, the budget, the Gantt chart, and the PERT network are examples of tools used both for planning and controlling. The flow chart, the flow process chart, the work distribution chart, and work sampling all may be used in planning workflow or assessing a proposed change in plan or procedure. They also may be adapted for specific control use, such as when the flow chart is employed to audit the way in which work is done, as compared to the original plan. Some control tools are directed at employee performance, such as the principle of requalification, discussed later in this chapter. Specific, quantifiable output measures may be recorded and monitored through a variety of visible control charts. In addition to these specific tools, the manager exercises control through the assessment and limitation of conflict, through the communication process, and through active monitoring of employees. These concepts were discussed in earlier chapters. Specific tools of planning and control are given here.

GANTT CHART

A visual control device, the Gantt chart was developed by Henry L. Gantt (1861–1919), one of the pioneers in scientific management. Sometimes referred to as a scheduling and progress chart, it emphasizes the work/time relationships necessary to meet some defined goal. The time needed for each activity is estimated, and a time value is assigned. This information is plotted on the chart. As the work progresses, entries are made to reflect the work completed. The chart focuses on the interrelationships among the phases of work within a given task. The Gantt chart may be used to reflect different aspects of the work:

1. machine or equipment scheduling (also called a load chart)
2. overall production control
3. individual worker production

Basic Components of Gantt Charts

The chart contains the same basic components, regardless of the application. The estimated time allotted for the work is plotted against a time scale that shows the appropriate time frame in days, weeks, or months, as well as calendar dates (Figure 10–1). The calendar legend may be placed at the top or bottom of the chart. As work progresses, items completed are entered and compared to those planned. In using the chart as a visual control tool, the manager uses shading or color coding to enter lines proportional in length to the percentage of work accomplished.

Figure 10-1 Gantt Progress Chart for Planning and Controlling Filing
Backlog: Laboratory Reports

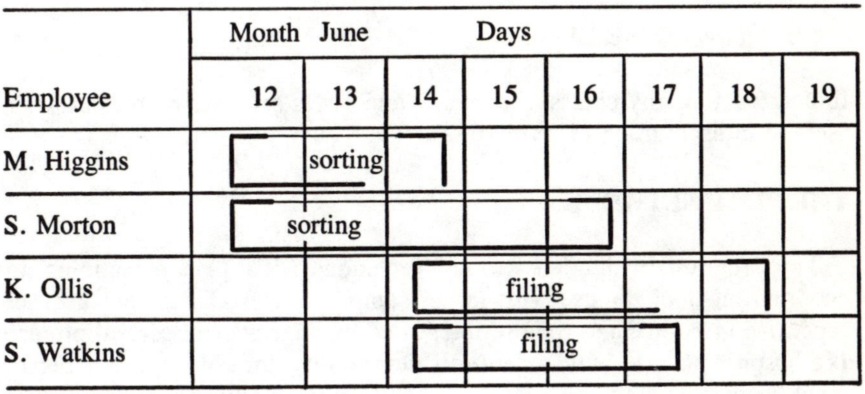

Employee	Month June Days							
	12	13	14	15	16	17	18	19
M. Higgins		sorting						
S. Morton	sorting							
K. Ollis				filing				
S. Watkins				filing				

Standard Symbols

Standard symbols are used for plotting the Gantt chart:

1. The "opening angle" is entered under the date an operation is planned to start.
2. The "closing angle" is entered under the date the operation is planned to be completed.
3. A straight line joining the opening and closing angle shows the time span within which the operation is to be done.
4. A heavy line shows work completed. This progress line usually is proportional to the amount of work completed.
5. A check mark is placed at the date when the progress was posted and is entered on the time scale.

An additional entry may show cumulative work done as time progresses. Codes may be entered to show the reason for being off schedule, such as

- W: worker unavailable due to illness or personal day
- M: lack of materials
- E: equipment breakdown

In constructing any charts, the legend and codes are entered for consistent use and interpretation (Figure 10–2).

THE PERT NETWORK

The Program Evaluation Review Technique (PERT) is a planning and coordinating tool for use with large, complex undertakings that are non-repetitive in nature and require integrated management of several projects. If a hospital plans to build an entirely new facility, for example, each department head must plan and coordinate the layout, equipment selection, work-flow determinations, and staffing patterns for the operations of his or her department. These, in turn, must be coordinated with the work of other departments. Other managers in the health care setting may face similar projects of a complex nature. An occupational therapist may be assigned to develop and implement a home care program within six months, a medical technologist may be assigned to oversee the conversion of several manual

Figure 10–2 Gantt Chart for Evaluating New Admissions

Therapist		Week 1						Week 2					
		M	T	W	Th	F	S-S	M	T	W	Th	F	S-S
A. Clay	AM		acute-2nd								W	W	Emerg. Acute
	PM												
D. Francis	AM							Acute admiss.					
	PM												
S. Scott	AM	W	W				Emerg. Acute-2nd						
	PM												
L. Matt	AM		Progress Update-staff										
	PM												
O. Rank	AM												
	PM												

laboratory techniques to a computerized system, a medical record administrator may face the task of converting 100,000 medical records from a serial filing system to a terminal digit system with unit record while maintaining the availability of records on a day-to-day basis, or a project manager must oversee the development of a fully operational quality assurance or risk management program by a specific date.

PERT's major components are the final goal statement, events to be accomplished, activities to be carried out, and critical time calculations to be monitored.

Historical Background

During the mid-1950s, the Department of the Navy's Special Projects Office determined that the Polaris missile system would constitute a critical element of U.S. defense. The work on the missile system involved approximately 9,000 subcontractors and 150,000 workers. A master planning and scheduling process was needed to reflect the work of the many aspects of this project.

Planning and controlling charts were in use in industry, but each had limitations. The Gantt chart, for example, was widely used in industry, but had an inherent limitation; while it shows relationships within tasks, it does not necessarily show relationships among all tasks. Although the Gantt chart shows progress along the projected time span for each activity, it cannot readily be determined if the task listed can be started before the successful completion of the previous task. For the Polaris project, a planning and controlling technique that reflected the dependent relationships of various aspects of the work was needed. The PERT network (Figure 10–3) was developed to show such relationships.

Advantages of Network Analysis

Seasoned experts at PERT network application caution the user not to spend more time on constructing the network than on carrying out the project. If the project is characterized by complex, nonrepetitive, interrelated activities, however, time probably is well spent on network construction; such detailed planning both permits and forces the manager to examine each major program and project in its entirety and in detail. The manager must identify and anticipate possible delays, which helps resolve difficulties. Network analysis enables the manager to identify deadlines that can be met ahead of schedule through the constant built-in monitoring aspect; consequently, the manager can save money, staff, and resources.

Figure 10-3 PERT Network: Conversion to In-House Transcription
Service

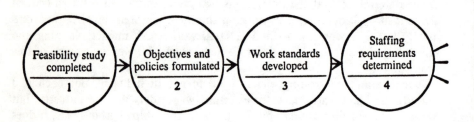

Figure 10-3 continued

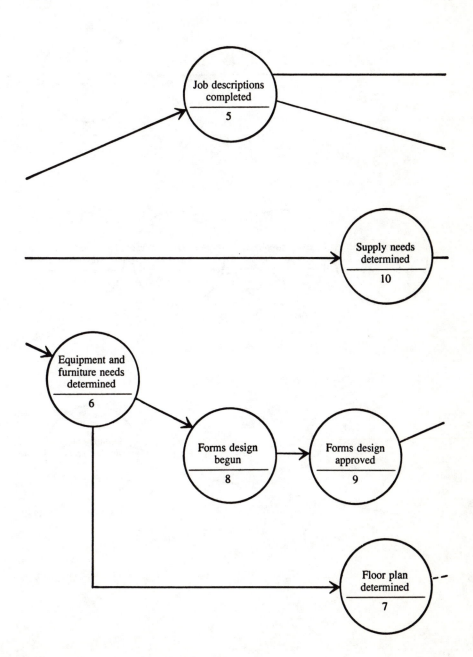

Figure 10–3 continued

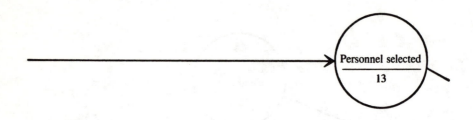

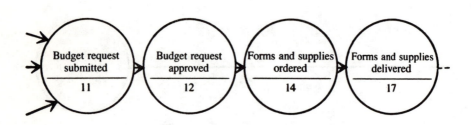

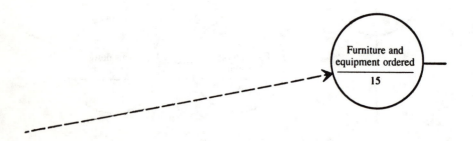

Figure 10–3 continued

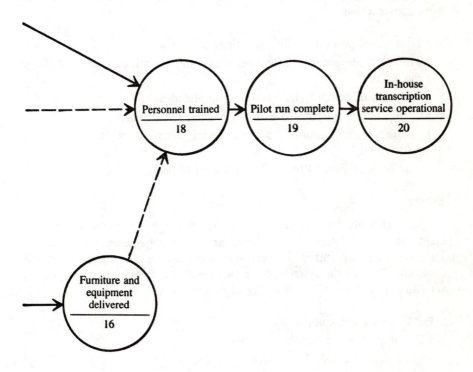

Fundamental Concepts

There are three phases in the PERT network: planning, scheduling, and controlling. These activities involve a specific goal that must be defined in detail. All events within the network and all activities performed flow from and are aimed toward accomplishment of this goal.

The Goal

The most basic concept in the PERT network is the statement of the goal. The network essentially is a diagrammatic representation of the plan for achieving this goal. The following are examples of goal statements for network construction:

- Home care program fully operational.
- Medical audit program fully operational in medical, surgical, and obstetrics units.
- Pilot test of computerized system completed.
- Conversion to automated laboratory system completed.
- Medical record storage system under terminal digit system fully operational.
- Nurses' aide trained to established level of performance.

Events

The work is divided into events so that the manager can check accomplishments against the plan. These events are the recognizable control points. They are discrete points in time and do not consume per se resources or time; they reflect either the starting or ending point for an activity or a group of activities. Examples of the wording of events are

- Job description completed.
- Training of home health aides begun.
- Computer selected.
- Renovation of storage area begun.
- Telephone system installed.

Although events are most frequently stated as work completed, the start of some events is a significant milestone. A network, therefore, contains both events stated as completed and events stated as begun. Events are depicted on the network by circles, rectangles, or ovals that contain the descriptive wording of the elements. Usually, events are numbered for ease of reference, but letters may be used if the number of events is limited. Figure 10–3 depicts events on a network, such as event 11 or event 12.

Certain events actually are subgoals in that no further activities and no additional events (except the final goal) flow from them. Such events are called "hanging events," because no other activities are needed to complete them. No successor event follows them, so they flow directly to the final goal.

Activities

An activity is defined as a recognizable part of a project that requires time and resources for its completion. Activities are the work necessary to progress from one event to another (i.e., from one point in time to another in the project schedule) and, ultimately, to the goal. These operations require time, money, resources, and staff. Activities connect events. The network is a diagrammatic representation of activities to be performed and events to be completed in terms of the goal to be reached. Normally, activities are depicted by a solid line between the events to which they are related. Activities are characterized by a specific initiating event, the *predecessor* event, and a specific terminal event, the *successor* event.

No descriptive wording is placed on the activity line. The activities are delineated in detail on an accompanying activity specification sheet, which includes the predecessor events, the successor events, and the responsible individuals (Exhibit 10–1). This facilitates, even forces, thorough planning. The wording of activities reflects their nature as work being done:

- developing job descriptions
- training home health aides
- selecting the computer
- renovating the storage area
- installing the telephone system

Exhibit 10–1 Activity Specification Sheet

Date _____
Predecessor event _____ Successor event_____
Activity name _____
Estimated time _____ Optimistic _____ Most likely _____ Pessimistic _____
Scheduled date _____ Completed date _____
Responsible individual _____
Specification of work:

The activities of a PERT network are read with the beginning and ending events as the reference point. Thus, the name of the activity as determined from the network refers to those specific elements involved in moving the plan from the beginning event to the desired state in the ending event. For example, given the following network

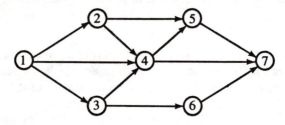

Table 10–1 shows the proper way of reading activities.

Table 10–1 Reading Activities on a PERT Network

Activity	Beginning Event	Ending Event
1–2	1	2
1–3	1	3
3–4	3	4
2–4	2	4
1–4	1	4
4–5	4	5

Interrelationships of Activities and Events

All activities and events in a program are related to each other in various ways. These relationships are called dependencies or constraints. Activities can be related to one another because they employ common resources; for example, those that must use the same facilities, equipment, or personnel and cannot do so concurrently are dependent on each other. Most dependency relationships result simply from the fact that a particular activity cannot begin until the product of the preceding action is available. In other words, certain events cannot occur until the previous one has been completed. Obviously, for example, a computer cannot be installed until after it has been selected. A merge event is one that is constrained immediately by two or more activities; a burst event is one constraining two or more activities. Large networks often contain many merge and burst events.

The following examples illustrate the interrelationship of activities and events, as well as the sequence of events.

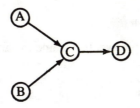

Event A = walls of building completed
Event B = walls of building painted
Event C = Special interior design completed

Thus, activity AB must be completed before activity BC can be started and completed.

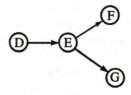

Event D = roof completed
Event E = siding completed
Event F = TV antenna installed
Event G = rainpipes installed

Thus, activity DE must be completed before either activity EF or activity EG can be started. It is not necessary to start activities EF and EG at the same time; the diagram simply emphasizes the relationship of event E to event F and that of event E to event G; if events F and G stood in some special relationship to one another, this would be shown through the use of the dummy or zero-time activity line.

In some cases, more than one event must be satisfied before a subsequent event can be started:

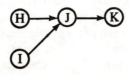

Both activities HJ and IJ must be completed before activity JK can be started. For example, an excavation must be completed and the building material received before construction can be started.

Dummy or Zero-Time Activities

The relationship between events in some instances is purely that of a constraint: no real activity occurs, no time is spent, no resource is consumed. This type of dependency is represented by a dummy or zero-time activity, which is usually depicted as a dotted or broken line rather than the solid line of a real activity. A network may contain a cluster of dummy activities as various subgoals are reached. Although no further activity occurs, it is necessary to show that the final goal is constrained by the preceding events. Dummy activities may also occur within the body of the network. The activity lines between events 16 and 18, and between events 17 and 18 illustrate dummy activities (Figure 10–3).

Figure 10–4 demonstrates the difference between real and dummy or zero-time activities. These examples are not from the same PERT network, nor are they related to each other; they are provided for emphasis. In the first example, budget requested and budget approved, many activities are involved. The activity specification sheet for this activity line typically includes such detailed elements as obtaining cost estimates for equipment, calculating salary increases for personnel, adjusting the budget after preliminary review, and merging unit budgets into a master budget. The time needed to complete these activities and the individuals responsible are stated on the activity specification sheet. The length of the activity line on the diagrammatic network is not necessarily proportional to the number of detailed activities nor to the amount of time needed to perform them. It is simply a matter of the mechanics of drawing the network and has no significance in itself.

Level of Indenture

The network is specific to the given program or project. The level of detail and degree of specificity should be custom-made for the project and should be consistent within the network. Highly detailed statements for some events and much more generalized statements for others create an imbalance. Because the network is first of all a planning tool, both the event statements and the activity specifications should be relatively specific. The planner may start with a gross network and refine it for greater specificity. Subnetworks may also be used for events that require a greater level of detail than that accorded most events in the network. Interface points are used on the master network to show the relationship points of the subnetworks. For control as the

Figure 10-4 Real vs. Zero-Time Activities

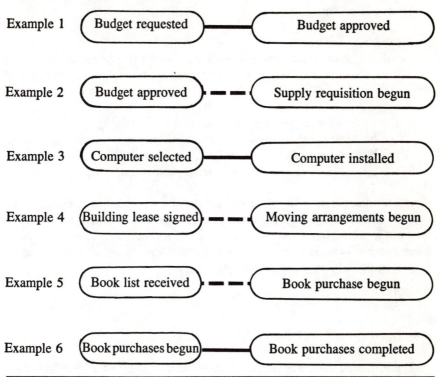

project is implemented, the manager needs to monitor specific and critical points; again, there is need for a consistent level of detail.

Use of Time Estimates

Because PERT involves control of projects after the planning stage is complete, it is necessary to estimate how long the project as a whole will take so that the manager can determine how much ahead of time or behind time it is at any given phase. Ordinarily, time in a PERT network is never estimated in units of less than a week, since most activities are of such magnitude that they take considerable time to accomplish. The Activity Specification Sheet (Exhibit 10-1) reveals the importance of time in that it includes the following terms related to time:

1. estimated time
2. optimistic
3. most likely

4. pessimistic
5. scheduled date
6. completed date

Usually, the individual with overall responsibility for an activity is involved in determining these times. Three estimates are obtained for each activity:

1. the worst (if everything goes wrong)—pessimistic, t_p
2. the best (no breakdown in equipment, no personnel turnover, no delay in obtaining materials)—optimistic, t_o
3. the probable (realistic considerations)—most likely, t_m

This assumes not only full-time utilization of given resources, but also successful completion of the predecessor event. At this point, the cumulative effect of a failure to complete predecessor events according to assigned deadlines can be seen. The manager actively monitors these deadlines, usually requiring periodic reporting of progress.

Constructing the PERT Network

The following steps are suggested in the construction of a PERT network:

1. State the final goal in detail. Then, work forward from beginning to end, stating all the events that must be completed to achieve the final goal; work backward from the goal to the beginning point; or use a combined approach.
2. List all possible events. It may be useful to write one event per card and work out the sequence later, sometimes best accomplished in a brainstorming session.
3. List activities. Although this is optional, it may help the manager differentiate activities from events or recall events to be specified.
4. Analyze events and place them in proper sequence. Look for critical relationships, logical flow, and dependencies.
5. Review the activities carefully to distinguish between real and dummy activities.
6. Remember that there may be a number of merge and burst events.
7. Diagram events and activities; number or letter the events.
8. Remember that the flow of activities and events is always forward; there are no backward loops in PERT.

The Critical Path

The expense of the overall project is of primary concern with the Critical Path Method network. Managers seek to reduce the cost by reducing the length of time required to accomplish the most time-consuming set of activities in the network. Managers assess the cost of a "crash" program and compare the increase in expense with the dollars saved if the goal is met earlier. If there is a saving, it is worthwhile to allot greater resources to critical activities. This approach is used commonly in construction projects. A similar technique is used in the field of manufacturing. The possibility of capturing the market ahead of a competitor sometimes makes it feasible to expend more money in reducing the critical path. This all ties in with probability, forecasting, and related techniques. At times, a particular outcome is vital, and attention to the critical path method may be warranted, even though specific dollars may not be saved.

THE FLOW CHART

The manager may use a flow chart to depict the chronological flow of work. A flow chart is a graphic representation of an ordered sequence of events, steps, or procedures that takes place in a system. The following are various types of flow charts:

- procedure flow chart: a graphic depiction of the distribution and subsequent steps in processing work.
- program block diagram: a detailed description of the steps that take place in computer routines. Specific operations and decisions, as well as their sequence in the program, are indicated.
- logic diagram: a graphic representation of the data-processing logic.
- two-dimensional flow chart: a depiction of complex workflow. This type of flow chart allows the procedures analyst to show a number of flows at the same time, such as a procedure that begins with a single action and branches out into several workflows (Figure 10–5).
- systems flow chart: a display of the information flow throughout all parts of the system. These flow charts may be task-oriented, i.e., may emphasize work performed, or they may be forms-oriented, i.e., may depict the flow of documents through the functional structure.

Flow charting is associated with computerized data processing because of its emphasis on logical flow, but it is not restricted to such program documentation. The flow chart may be used to advantage by any manager who must analyze, plan, and control workflow.

Figure 10–5 Two-Dimensional Flow Chart

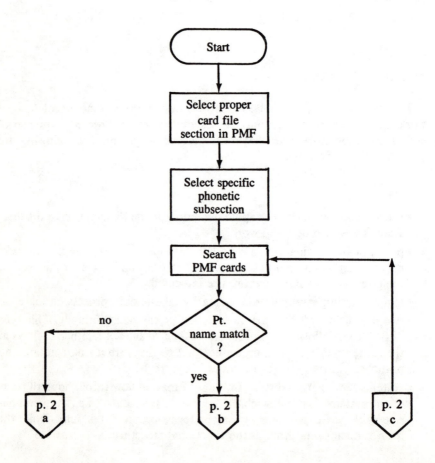

Figure 10–5 continued

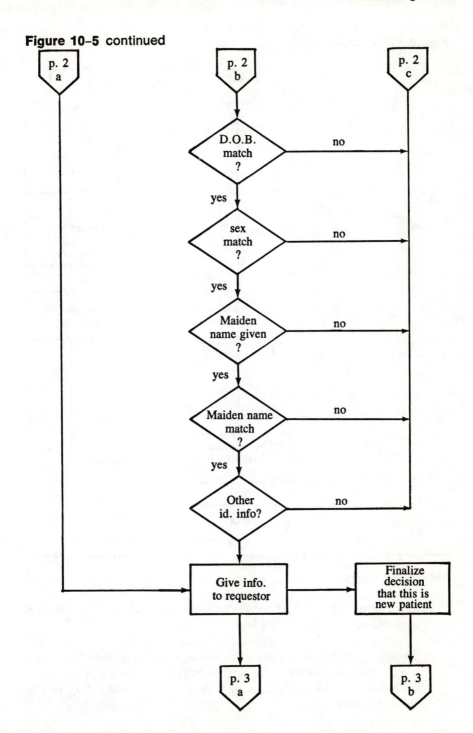

Figure 10-5 continued

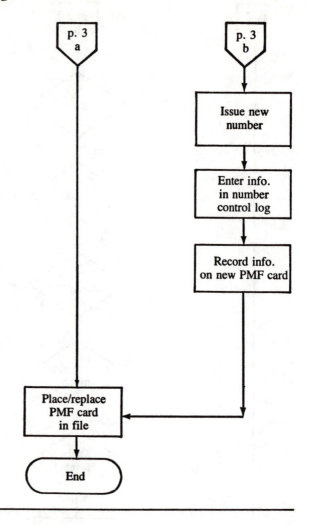

___

Uses of the Flow Chart

The flow chart may be used for both planning and controlling activities. As a planning tool, it may be used to

1. develop a procedure. It forces the manager to think logically, since it reveals how one aspect of the task is linked to others, which areas of workflow must be made consistent, and where coordination mechanisms are needed.

2. illustrate and emphasize key points in the written procedure. The flow chart may be used as companion documentation to the written procedure, as it provides an overall picture of the workflow in concise form. Key points in the workflow may be emphasized by color coding critical decisions or actions.
3. compare present and proposed procedures. A comparison of a flow chart for a proposed procedure with a flow chart for the existing procedure may show that there are as many, or more, delays in the proposed procedure.

It is less costly to assess the probable outcome of a procedure before it is implemented than to find that the procedure is not workable after it has been implemented.

As a control device, the flow chart may be used to

1. compare the actual workflow with that originally planned. In order to remain effective guides to actions, procedures must be updated and the workflow must be monitored for changes that occur imperceptibly. By developing a flow chart of current practice and comparing it with the original plan, the manager can see changes that have occurred in the workflow and may then decide whether to change the procedure so that it reflects existing practice or to enforce compliance with the original procedure.
2. audit the workflow. Every loop in a flow chart is a potential delay; the manager can pinpoint areas of delay, investigate the legitimacy of the delays, and determine how to shorten or eliminate them.

Flow Chart Symbols

On a flow chart, each distinctive symbol stands for a certain kind of function, such as decision making, processing, or input-output. Symbols provide a shorthand method of describing the processes involved in the work. These symbols, which have become standardized in data processing, are used for flow charts in connection with both computer programs and with noncomputerized systems analysis. Commonly accepted flow chart symbols are shown in Figure 10–6.

Figure 10–6 Flow Chart Symbols

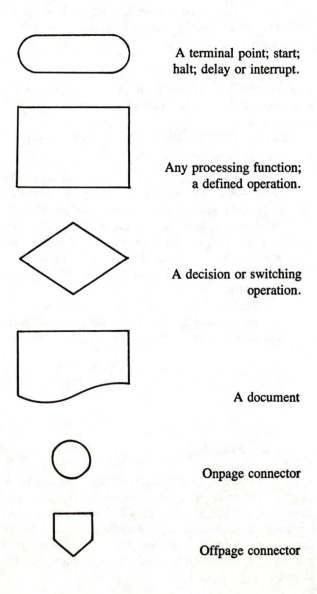

A terminal point; start; halt; delay or interrupt.

Any processing function; a defined operation.

A decision or switching operation.

A document

Onpage connector

Offpage connector

Support Documentation

Sometimes the flow chart is a companion document to a fully written procedure. When the flow chart depicts the overall systems flow or when the procedure has not yet been developed, support documentation is needed to complement the information on the chart. This documentation may be in the form of notes in the body of the flowchart or in the form of a narrative statement. Notes are brief, clarifying statements that supply information in conjunction with a process. They are keyed to their proper place in the chart by a number or a letter. Notes are placed in side or bottom margins where they will not interfere with the flow chart proper. A narrative statement covers assumptions, questions, and areas that need additional follow-up. A brief summary of the overall setting of the workflow may be included. Any special terms or abbreviations used are defined in this document.

THE FLOW PROCESS CHART

Sometimes referred to simply as a process chart, the flow process chart is a graphic representation of events that depicts the chronological flow of work or a product through an entire workflow cycle or through some part of it. Each detail of the workflow is clearly recorded with the appropriate symbols; each step can be questioned and analyzed to identify areas for possible improvement.

The flow process chart may be developed to present the process in terms of the material flow or in terms of the activity of the workers. The specific focus, material or worker, must be decided at the beginning of the study, information about the material and the worker cannot be recorded on the same chart. Should information on both aspects of the work be needed, two separate charts must be developed.

Flow Process Chart vs. Flow Chart

Although both are graphic representations of the workflow, the flow process chart differs from the flow chart. The symbols used to record the information are different for the two charts, and the information recorded and made available for analysis differs in its emphasis. The flow process chart contains specific entries for time units, distances, and qualities; it also contains specific questions for step-by-step analysis (Figure 10–7). On the flow chart, in contrast, this information is shown in supplementary notes; furthermore, it is not gathered as precisely as it is in the flow process chart. In addition, the flow process chart does not have the branching capability of the flow chart; simultaneous flow of work must be shown on separate flow process charts and cross-referenced by special notes.

Figure 10-7 Flow Process Chart

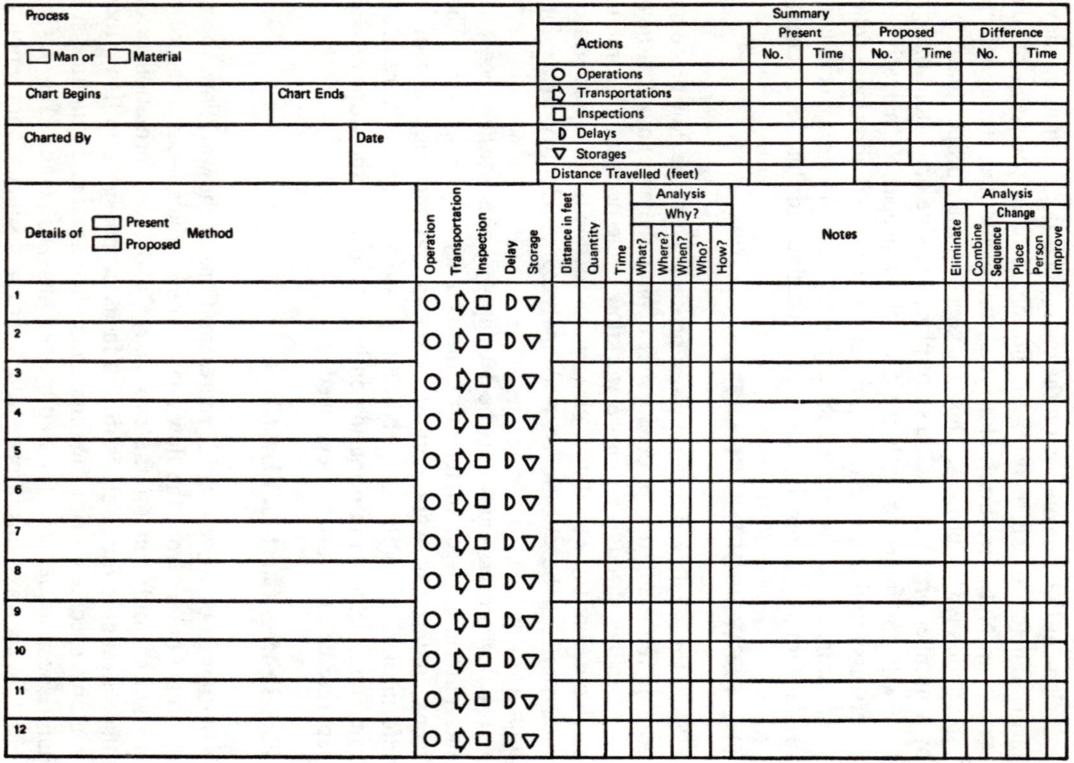

The flow process chart permits the recording of information in great detail, which is both an advantage and a limitation. The mass of details may be so great that it becomes excessively time-consuming to analyze the results properly. Also, information on the flow process chart may be distorted, especially when the focus is on the material. Reasons for apparent delays must be carefully analyzed. For example, a laboratory requisition slip may be placed in a temporary file while the results are being obtained; this appears as a delay, although important activity is occurring.

Uses of the Flow Process Chart

The flow process chart is used to break down and analyze individual operations in detail in order to

1. develop and verify procedures
2. compare present and proposed procedures
3. obtain specific information about time factors and delays in operations, as well as about distance factors in transportation and work movement
4. analyze workflow to improve procedures by eliminating overlap and minimizing delays
5. assess physical layout with emphasis on (a) transportation distance between equipment and work station and (b) relationship of one work station to another
6. gather information to use with other data to set work standards, especially when delay and transportation are factors
7. establish a basis for further study, such as detailed analyses of bottlenecks in the workflow, excessive delays, and backtracking

Standard Symbols

The standard symbols for flow process chart usage are those endorsed by the Administrative Management Society and the American Society of Mechanical Engineers (Figure 10–8).

Operation

An operation occurs when an object is changed in any of its physical characteristics, when information is given or received, when planning or calculation takes place, or when a worker carries out an activity. Operations are the main steps in a process. The end result is usually something produced or accomplished; something is being done to or by the subject, or something is being created, changed, or added to. The symbol for an operation is a large circle O. Unshaded, this symbol is used for nonproductive activities, such as

Figure 10-8 Approved Flow Process Chart Symbols

Symbol	Element
◯	Operation
⇨	Transportation
▽	Storage
□	Inspection
D	Delay

make ready or put away operations (e.g., sort appointment cards, arrange orders in account number sequence, or pick up medications). Shaded, the operation symbol shows a "do" or productive operation, such as clean a needle, type a letter, or fill in monthly rates.

Transportation

Except when the movement is a part of the operation or is caused by the operator at the work station during an operation or inspection, movement of an object from one place to another is considered a transportation process. The symbol for transportation is an arrow ⇨. Examples of transportation processes are appointment slip carried to work area, medication card carried to medication cabinet, empty trays returned to cart, and supplies carried to table. A letter placed in the outbasket is an operation, while a letter carried to the mailroom (from one work station to another) is a transportation process. The distance travelled is usually included on the chart as supplementary information in conjunction with the transportation process.

Storage

When an object is kept, protected against unauthorized removal, and made available for future use, it is in its authorized storage place. The object is disposed of permanently, or it remains in one place for a period of time awaiting further action. The symbol for storage is the inverted triangle ▽. Examples of storage include medical record placed in permanent file, medications stored in cabinet at nurses' station, reagents placed in bottle, or medication card put in medication card file until next medication is given.

Inspection

During an inspection, an object is examined for identification or verified for quality or quantity in any of its characteristics. Objects are checked, verified, reviewed, or examined, but no change is made. The symbol for inspection is the square □. Examples of inspection include appointment slip scanned by clerk for patient identification, letter proofread, and medication compared to master medication sheet entry by nurse.

Delay

When conditions do not permit or require immediate performance of the next planned action, a person or object is interrupted or delayed in flow. Such actions as placing an object in temporary storage, e.g., in a desktop file, where it awaits the next action are included in the concept of delay. A delay is shorter in duration than storage. The symbol for delay is a stylized **D**. Examples of delay include a wait by a nurse while medications are taken by the patient, a letter in an outbox waiting for pickup, a patient's wait to visit a clinic, a worker's wait for an elevator, equipment awaiting transportation, and appointment slips placed in a chronological file. A standard unit of time measure, e.g., minutes, is usually included.

Factors outside the Study

Certain outside influences that temporarily disrupt the workflow may be outside the scope of a designated study. If the analyst considers some process impractical to evaluate, it is noted as an outside interference, usually of a temporary nature. An elevator may be broken, causing more than usual delay; an area may be under renovation; or equipment may not function properly. Should this influencing factor be noted repeatedly, the manager should take some corrective action; should it be beyond the control of the manager, it should be taken into account in the assessment of overall constraints on the workflow. To determine which of the elements in the process is involved in such a constraint, it is useful to review them in terms of the intent of these definitions of standards symbols:

Element/Process	Intent
Operation	Produces or accomplishes
Transportation	Moves
Inspection	Verifies
Delay	Interferes
Storage	Keeps

Flow Process Chart Format

The form typically used for a flow process chart contains standard elements of information, although these elements may be arranged in different ways. After the header information has been completed, the body of the flow process chart is developed:

1. Step numbers are listed chronologically, and numbers are assigned to each step for easy reference in the note section or in the related narrative documentation.
2. Events are described as briefly as possible, but clearly. It is helpful to use the active voice when describing the worker's movement, e.g., fill out medication card; passive voice when describing the flow of material, e.g., medication card filled out.
3. The appropriate symbol for each step in the process is determined and entered in a column reserved for that entry.
4. Supplemental information, such as distance in feet, quantity, or time, is entered. This is tallied and summarized after all the data have been gathered for the entire workflow under study.
5. Analysis questions are raised as part of the review of the workflow. These may be simply checked off and analyzed in detail as a separate step. The questions are straightforward: who? what? when? how? where?
6. Space is provided to make special notes, such as cross-references to a previous step, additional factors to be examined, or factors in the physical layout.
7. Action questions concerning possible change are included: eliminate the step? combine? improve sequence, place, person? These action questions are combined with the analytical questions.

Space is provided for a summary section, which contains a tabulation of the various operational steps or elements. Space is also provided to enter the totals for time spent and distance travelled. Data for the present and proposed methods may be included, as well as a calculation of the differences in the two methods.

Steps in Developing Flow Process Chart

The usual steps to develop a flow process chart are summarized here for review and reference:

1. choose the job to be studied; be specific

2. refine the focus of the study by selecting
   a. the subject to be studied, person or material, present or proposed method
   b. the starting and stopping point of the study
3. complete identification section of the chart
4. list each step in sequence and enter any explanatory notes in the appropriate column
5. apply the correct symbol for each activity; be consistent in use of accepted symbols. Shade the productive operations to highlight those activities.
6. enter time, distance, and quantity where appropriate. Use consistent units to enter these data (e.g., inches or feet, seconds or minutes).
7. draw a line to connect each symbol to emphasize the idea of the flow of the work
8. summarize the findings; enter the figures in the appropriate spaces

THE WORK DISTRIBUTION CHART

Although their overall goals may remain constant, organizations are in a state of continual change. Therefore, continual monitoring of the organizational structure is needed. If the actual distribution of work shifts from the original workflow plan, the manager must determine whether the present distribution of work among the organizational units is an improvement. If so, the structure should be adjusted; if not, appropriate measures should be taken to restore the original workflow plan and the original organizational structure.

One managerial tool for gathering factual data about the present organizational system is the work distribution chart, which focuses on work assignments and job content within any single unit or work group. This chart is designed to show (1) major activities of the unit, (2) total hours (per standard time period) spent on each activity, and (3) total hours (per standard time period) spent by each worker on each task. If the chart has been properly prepared, it shows the

1. amount of time spent on each activity
2. degree of specialization
3. overlap in work distribution
4. fragmentation in work
5. uneven distribution of work

This information must be analyzed to determine whether the degree of specialization is adequate or excessive; whether the amount of time is appropriate, excessive, or disproportionate to the significance of the activity; whether the fragmentation is unavoidable or is the result of overspecialization; and whether some employees are overloaded while others lack work.

The purpose of the work distribution chart is to gather information in a consistent manner and to display this information in a way that facilitates critical review (Figure 10–9). It is customary to list workers in descending order by job rank. Name and job title are placed along the horizontal plane, left to right. Major activities and time tallies are listed in vertical columns.

The work distribution chart is prepared by the unit supervisor or manager from the information contained in the daily task lists (Exhibit 10–2) kept by each worker. The daily task list is a record of the time each worker spends each working day on each activity. The manager develops the basic form and gives the appropriate instructions to the staff, emphasizing that work distribution studies are not used for employee evaluation and that the focus is on the distribution of the work, not personal productivity.

The manager provides a list of definitions for each activity so that the usage of terms is consistent. Instructions are also given as to the time units to be used, usually segments of 15 minutes. It is not necessary, however, to account for every minute. The idle times, rest periods, and delays could be grouped under the miscellaneous category. If that category's total seems

---

Exhibit 10–2 Daily Task List

Employee:	Date: _____
Job Title:	

Time Period	Task Performed

Figure 10-9 Work Distribution Chart: Medical Records Division

Department: Medical Records

Week of May 14 to May 18

Unit: Correspondance

ACTIVITY	Total Hours (all employees)	Agusta Bernard Supervisor	Hours	Laura Case Clerk II	Hours	Martha Cossian Clerk I	Hours
Telephone Requests	8		1		3		4
In-Person Requests	14		11		3		
Subpoena/ Depositions	12	* Prepare charts * Attend court sessions	12				
Obtaining Patient ID for requests	6					* Checking patient master file	6
Chart Retrieval	11			* Complete chargeout cards * Retrieve charts	1		10
Abstracting Reply	42		10		26		6
Photocopying	7					* Daily Photocopying	7
Miscellaneous	20	* Supervisor's Meeting * Session with trainees	4 2	* Emergency coverage in files 5/15	7	* File area coverage 5/16	7
TOTAL	120		40		40		40

unusually high (above the customary 10 to 15 percent allowed for personal, fatigue, and delay factors in work standards and time studies), a separate investigation should be done.

The supervisor or manager collects the daily task lists and compiles the summary task list for each worker in the unit. These summary task lists are assembled at the end of some predetermined period, e.g., at the end of a work week (Exhibit 10–3). In constructing the work distribution chart, the manager follows the customary rules for conducting a work study, such as consistency in gathering facts, selection of a representative work period, and inclusion of the entire work cycle.

Exhibit 10–3 Weekly Task List

Employee:	Week of _____
Job Title:	
Tasks Performed	**Hours**

BIBLIOGRAPHY

Archibold, Russell D. *Network-Based Management Systems* (PERT/CPM). New York: John Wiley & Sons, 1967.

Bettersby, Albert. *Network Analysis for Planning and Scheduling.* New York: St. Martin's Press, 1964.

Levin, Richard, and Kirkpatrick, Charles. *Planning and Control with PERT/CPM.*

Lott, Richard. *Basic Systems Analysis.* San Francisco: Canfield Press, 1971.

Chapter 11

Work Sampling

CHAPTER OBJECTIVES

1. Define work sampling.
2. Relate work sampling to the control process.
3. Cite uses of work sampling.
4. Relate the concept of random sampling to work sampling.
5. Apply the use of alignment charts, random number tables, and observation tables to departmental work sampling.

Work may be measured by means of several approaches, such as stopwatch studies, micromotion studies, and work sampling. The technique of work sampling, i.e., making a series of observations at random intervals, is based on the statistical principle that observations made at random provide information as complete as that provided by a continuous method of time study. Work sampling is sometimes called ratio delay, as it was developed in the British textile industry where the ratio of delays to productive work was determined through a process of random observations.

The technique consists of periodic, but frequent, spot checks of the worker, the equipment, or the activity; the observations are recorded and then analyzed. Specific uses of work sampling include

- determining downtime on a machine

- identifying patterns of delay or interference in the workflow

- verifying job content; comparing job duties assigned or originally described with actual job content

- determining discrepancies in workflow between what was planned and what is occurring

- determining what percentage of the workday is spent on each job or activity
- determining what percentage of an overall job is done by each worker
- establishing delay factors in setting work standards

The work sampling technique allows the manager or observer to carry out the study while concurrently doing other work, since it is not a continuous time study (as is a stopwatch study). Work sampling is relatively inexpensive to do and may be carried out by a nonstatistical practitioner. Because the content is closely related to other managerial data, the major items for study are readily identifiable. For example, the job description lists the major duties of a worker, task assignment records contain the major worker assignments, and systems and workflow statements contain details of the planned work.

The work sampling technique is best suited for the study of jobs with a few major tasks. Limits of the technique include the possibility of worker tendency to perform when under observation and the possibility of observer bias in developing the study and carrying out the observations. These problems can be overcome by adherence to the underlying principles of sampling, however. The observations should be made at random, rather than casually or haphazardly. The worker should be informed that the study is a series of observations to evaluate the work process, not employee performance. The study should be carried out over a period of time long enough so that the worker becomes accustomed to being observed and becomes relatively unaware of the process. The sample size should be representative, and the degree of precision or confidence level of the study should be sufficiently high to give validity to the study. The observation period should reflect a suitable work cycle that includes both peak load and off cycles in the work.

KEY CONCEPTS

Work sampling is based on the statistical principle of probability or "the law of averages." The following are key terms:

- *population* or *universe:* all the things of a kind in which one is interested; the subject of the study, such as all the beans in a jar, all the patients in the outpatient clinic, all the students in a class, all the employees of a department, all the residents in long-term care facilities for the mentally retarded
- *sample:* a small part of the population or universe, intended to reflect or represent the quality or nature of the whole, such as a handful of beans

from the jar, a few patients from the outpatient clinic, some of the students in a class

- *random:* the condition that exists when every element of the population has the same probability of being selected as part of the sample

The basic law of statistical probability is based on the premise that a small sample, selected at random from the given population, tends to reflect the same pattern and to have the same distribution as the whole.

Random sampling is commonly illustrated by visualizing a container of black and white marbles. Given a container of well-mixed black and white marbles, and given the information that 50 of the marbles are black and 50 of the marbles are white, there is a 50-50 chance of pulling either a black or a white marble from the container. Each time a marble is pulled, its color is noted; after it has been returned to the container and the marbles mixed, additional marbles are pulled to complete the sample number. Returning the marble to the container after noting its color is termed "sampling with replacement," a technique that allows the researcher to approximate an infinite population. Failure to replace the pulled marble alters the mix of colors and changes the odds as to which color will be drawn next.

The larger the sample size (the more times a marble is drawn from the container), the more closely the sample results approach the true percentage in the population or universe of the study. On only 3 draws, for example, the percentage of one color marble might be as high as 100 percent; as more draws are made, such as 20 draws, the sample results may show 55 percent of one color being drawn, which more closely reflects the equal mix of the sample.

SELECTION OF SAMPLE SIZE

The size of the sample selected is a function of statistical calculation and common sense. The sample must be large enough to reflect the universe to be studied, but not so large that it will be unwieldy, time-consuming, and expensive to analyze. It is costly to carry out a large sample and it may be unnecessary, depending on the purpose of the study. The analyst must choose a sample that is large enough to be valid and small enough to be economical. Sample size is also dependent on the desired degree of accuracy. The analyst must determine the level of confidence that is desirable for the study. Usually, a 95 percent confidence interval is used. The width of such an interval is defined by placing 1.96 standard deviation units around the arithmetic mean or average. In effect, the analyst is accepting a 5 percent error on either side of the results. "Give or take 5 times out of a hundred, the following results are accurate" summarizes the implication of a 95 percent confidence interval. Given a group of random observations, the results will be correct 95 percent of the time; stated another way, the results will be incorrect only 5 percent of the time.

Statistical formulas are available to calculate sample size. As a shortcut for the nonstatistical practitioner, alignment charts can be used to calculate the number of observations required to achieve a specific level of precision at a given confidence level. Figure 11–1 is an alignment chart that can be used for all 95 percent confidence levels. To use the alignment chart, several steps must be followed. The analyst must estimate the time spent on the job element; this information would be obtained from past records, common sense observations, and rough sampling of observations.

Column A of the alignment chart shows the element to be measured by listing percent of the work constituted by the element. In this example, the major tasks were roughly assessed through 64 observations. Of these, 51 showed that the major duties constituted the bulk of the work, as had been planned in the original division of the work. Dividing 51 by 64 gives 80 percent as the percent for the element to be measured. This 80 is plotted on the chart by aligning a straight edge at 80.

The next step involves choosing the desired precision. For example, if the maximum deviation allowed is to be 4 percentage points of 80 percent (80% ± 4%), 4 percent is plotted on the precision interval scale of column B. A straight edge is aligned so that it crosses through the 80 percent in column A and through the 4 percent in column B.

Extension of the line connecting columns A and B over to column C indicates the number of observations required for 95 percent accuracy on a major job constituting 80 percent of the activities or elements to be measured. The number of observations needed in this example is 400.

By way of further illustration in the use of the alignment chart, determine the number of observations needed for 95 percent accuracy in the following example:

> Given a major activity that constitutes 80 percent of the job and a desire to be within 1.6 percentage points of 80 percent (80% ± 1.6%), align the straight edge at 80 in column A, locate and plot 1.6 percent in column B, and construct a line to column C. A total of about 2,500 observations would be needed. The statistical formula for this calculation is illustrated in Exhibit 11–1. A nomogram is developed through a series of such statistical calculations.

Clearly, the smaller the error tolerance, the larger the sample size must be.

Figure 11-1 Alignment Chart

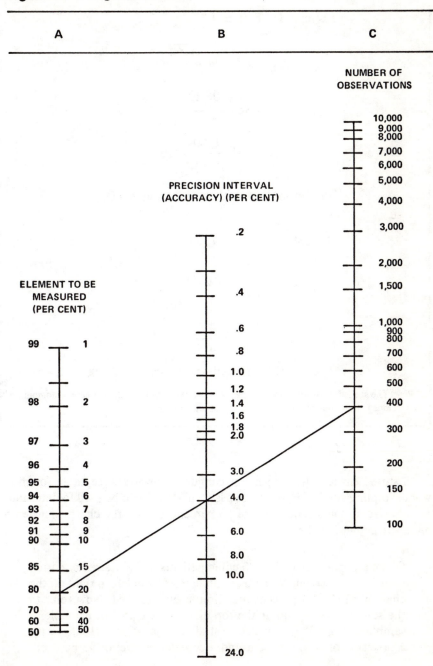

Figure 11-1 continued

Example 1:   80% ± 4%

$$80 \pm 1.96 \frac{\sqrt{p \times q}}{n}$$

$$1.96 \frac{\sqrt{80 \times 20}}{n} = 4$$

$$3.8416 \frac{1600}{(n)} = 16$$

n = 384 – plotted on nomogram at 400

Example 2:   92% ± 1.6%

$$1.96 \left(\frac{\sqrt{92 \times 8}}{n} \right) = 1.6$$

$$3.8416 \frac{736}{(n)} = 2.56$$

n = 1104 – plotted on nomogram at 1,200

Note: The statistical formula for calculation of sample size is illustrated here; a nomogram is developed through a series of such statistical calculations.

As stated earlier, the 95 percent confidence level is acceptable for most work sampling studies. Exhibit 11–1 is a chart that can be used to determine sample size at confidence levels of 95 percent. To use the chart, first determine the population size:

Given a population of 10,000 clinic patients and a desired precision within ± 4.4 percent of the true value, read from left to right on the chart until the 4.4 percent precision level is located. Now refer to the sample size legend at the top of the chart. In this example, a sample size of 500 is required to study a population of 10,000 with a precision of ± 4.4 percent and a confidence level of 95 percent.

Exhibit 11-1 Sample Size Calculation*

Population Size				Sample Size				
	400	450	500	750	1,000	1,250	1,500	2,000
200								
300								
400								
500	2.2	1.5						
600	2.9	2.4	1.8					
700	3.3	2.8	2.4					
800	3.5	3.1	2.7	0.9				
900	3.7	3.3	3.0	1.5				
1,000	3.9	3.5	3.2	1.8				
2,000	4.5	4.1	3.9	2.9	2.2	1.7	1.3	
3,000	4.7	4.3	4.1	3.2	2.6	2.1	1.8	1.3
4,000	4.7	4.4	4.2	3.3	2.7	2.3	2.0	1.6
5,000	4.8	4.5	4.2	3.4	2.8	2.4	2.2	1.7
10,000	4.9	4.6	4.4	3.5	3.0	2.6	2.4	2.0
25,000	5.0	4.7	4.4	3.6	3.1	2.8	2.5	2.1
50,000	5.0	4.7	4.4	3.6	3.1	2.8	2.6	2.2
100,000	5.0	4.7	4.4	3.6	3.1	2.8	2.6	2.2
200,000	5.0	4.7	4.4	3.6	3.1	2.8	2.6	2.2
300,000	5.0	4.7	4.5	3.6	3.2	2.8	2.6	2.2
400,000	5.0	4.7	4.5	3.6	3.2	2.8	2.6	2.2
500,000	5.0	4.7	4.5	3.6	3.2	2.8	2.6	2.2
1,000,000	5.0	4.7	4.5	3.7	3.5	2.8	2.6	2.2
2,000,000	5.0	4.7	4.5	3.7	3.5	2.8	2.6	2.2
3,000,000	5.0	4.7	4.5	3.7	3.5	2.8	2.6	2.2
4,000,000	5.0	4.7	4.5	3.7	3.5	2.8	2.6	2.2
5,000,000	5.0	4.7	4.5	3.7	3.5	2.8	2.6	2.2
10,000,000	5.0	4.7	4.5	3.7	3.5	2.8	2.6	2.2

INTERVAL SAMPLING

Certain aspects of work may be assessed by means of interval sampling, a technique in which the specific elements to be studied in the total population are determined through the use of an interval fraction. Work activities in a hospital that are suitable for interval sampling include the following:

- Given 10,000 medical records per week to be refiled accurately, how many records were returned to proper location?

- Given an average of 16,000 outpatient visits per month, how many patients' records have appropriate progress note entries?

- Given 630 laboratory studies per week, how many were left incomplete because of an inaccurate specimen draw?

The first example is described in detail to illustrate the use of interval sampling. A sample of 500 records is to be drawn from the population of 10,000 refiled records:

1. Calculate the average number of charts to be refiled per week; in this example, 10,000 is the total population of the study.
2. Calculate the sample size (see earlier discussion of sample size): in this case, 500 charts will be checked for proper location.
3. Calculate the interval by dividing the total population (10,000 records per week) by the sample size (500):

$$\frac{10,000}{500} = 20$$

This gives an interval of 20, or the selection of every 20th element from the total population in the study.
4. Select the starting point by choosing a random number between 1 and 20. Use the random number table or a calculator to obtain this number. In this example, the random number table in Exhibit 11-2 was consulted. Random entry into the chart was at the second batch of numbers on the right hand side, precisely at the second line of numbers: 52 53 37 97 15. The number 15 was the first usable one accessed.

Therefore, beginning with the 15th record returned, every 20th record returned in the study week is checked to determine if it has reached its proper location in the file. Numbers studied are 15, 35, 55, 75, 95, etc.

To carry out this particular study, the chargeout/tracer forms must be saved for the week so that it can be determined which medical records were returned that week. The analyst in the study must anticipate such a need and take the necessary steps.

SELECTION OF OBSERVATION TIMES

In selecting observation times, the manager must take into account the work cycle and the workday/hours within a weekly or monthly work cycle. If a total of 800 observations must be made over one month of working days (weekends omitted), 40 observations per day must be made (800 observations divided by 20 working days). This cycle of a full month of working days allows the manager to sample the work without subjecting the worker to intense observation on any one workday and without missing important variables in the workday as it is influenced by the flow of work throughout a month's cycle of activity.

Specific times in the workday must be chosen for making the observations, and these times should be selected randomly. One way is to write each time on a slip, mix all the slips, place them in a box, and choose the times for each day's observations from all the times in the box. This process can be cumbersome and time-consuming, however.

Random Number Tables

In random number tables, sequences of numbers are displayed in such a way that it is just as likely for any given digit, 0 through 9, to follow any other given digit. This is true whether the path for number selection is horizontal, vertical, or diagonal. Random number tables are used to draw a truly random sample (Exhibit 11–2). Such tables may be found in standard form in compilations of statistical tables. Some calculators have a random number function, which is another source of random number generation.

The table is consulted in a random manner. The user simply opens to some page in the random number table and accepts the first digit or set of digits displayed. The number is recorded on a work sheet, and additional numbers are taken from the random number table and recorded until sufficient usable numbers have been selected. If the table in Exhibit 11–2 is entered randomly, for example, the second block of numbers on the extreme left of the table might be chosen. Accepting the numbers as given, the user would find the following three-digit numbers by reading from left to right across the chart:

630	173
206	430
344	734

Exhibit 11–2 Section of a Random Number Table

91	76	21	64	60	94	21	78	55	09	55	34	57	92	69
00	97	79	08	06	34	41	92	45	71	69	66	92	19	09
36	40	18	34	94	53	14	30	59	25	86	96	98	29	06
88	98	99	60	50	88	59	53	11	52	90	92	10	70	80
04	37	69	87	21	65	28	04	67	53	74	16	32	23	02
63	02	06	34	41	73	43	07	34	48	16	95	86	70	75
78	47	23	53	90	48	62	11	90	60	52	53	37	97	15
87	68	62	19	43	28	97	85	58	99	56	61	87	33	12
47	60	92	10	77	02	63	45	52	38	21	94	47	90	12
56	88	87	59	41	76	96	59	38	72	23	32	65	41	18
02	57	45	86	67	79	88	01	51	48	26	29	13	56	41
31	54	14	13	17	08	25	58	94	43	77	80	20	75	82
28	50	10	43	36	84	99	87	40	75	46	40	66	44	52
63	29	62	66	50	36	37	34	92	09	61	65	81	98	60
45	65	58	26	51	01	16	96	65	27	93	69	64	43	07

The randomness of the table must not be destroyed by starting on the same page and in the same place each time. The odds are against this, unless the book is so well-worn that it opens often to the same page. Another potential distortion in the use of the random number table results from the tendency to read only from left to right. Numbers may also be selected by reading up and down, right to left, diagonally, and so forth.

One way of developing observation times with the use of a random number table is given by Ralph Barnes.[1] The first digit of a number taken from the table might indicate the hour of the day; the second and third digits, the minutes. Thus, if the number taken from the table is 950622, 950 would indicate 9.50, which is 9:30 (0.50 equals one-half of 60 minutes, or half past the hour). The second number 622 might indicate 6.22, or approximately 6:13 (0.22 of 60 minutes, or 13 minutes past the hour). If the company hours are 8:00 A.M. to 5:00 P.M., the number 6.22 would be discarded, and the next random number listed on the table would be selected and translated into a time of day. The manager continues this process until the desired total of observation times for the day has been obtained.

Observation Table

In an observation table, each minute in a workday is listed and a number assigned to that minute. For example, on Exhibit 11–3, the tenth minute of this workday is 8:39 (010). An observation table may be used in conjunction with a random number table to select observation times.

The following is a detailed example of the use of the random number table (Exhibit 11–2) in conjunction with the observation table (Exhibit 11–3):

1. Select numbers from the random number table, starting at the same point as used earlier.

630	867	605
206	075	253
344	784	379
173	723	715
430	539	876
734	048	862
481	621	194
695	190	etc.

2. Because this observation table spans the numbers 001 to 480, only these and any other numbers that fall between them may be used. Numbers above 480 are discarded for this study. Should the manager wish to carry the work study into workhours beyond 4:30, the observation table would be adjusted accordingly (e.g., 481 would indicate 4:31 P.M.). Discard any numbers above 480.

Exhibit 11–3 Observation Table: 8:30 A.M. to 4:30 P.M. Workday

001	8:30	016	8:45	031	9:00	046	9:15
002	8:31	017	8:46	032	9:01	047	9:16
003	8:32	018	8:47	033	9:02	048	9:17
004	8:33	019	8:48	034	9:03	049	9:18
005	8:34	020	8:49	035	9:04	050	9:19
006	8:35	021	8:50	036	9:05		
007	8:36	022	8:51	037	9:06		
008	8:37	023	8:52	038	9:07	Such an ob-	
009	8:38	024	8:53	039	9:08	servation ta-	
010	8:39	025	8:54	040	9:09	ble would	
011	8:40	026	8:55	041	9:10	continue in	
012	8:41	027	8:56	042	9:11	this manner	
013	8:42	028	8:57	043	9:12	through 480,	
014	8:43	029	8:58	044	9:13	that is, 4:30	
015	8:44	030	8:59	045	9:14	P.M.	

3. Arrange the remaining numbers in numerical order:

> 048
> 075
> 173
> etc.

4. Correlate the numbers with the times of day given in the observation chart:

> 048 = 9:17
> 075 = 9:44
> 173 = 11:22
> etc.

5. Enter the numbers in the column for "Observation Time" on the work sampling record form (Exhibit 11–4).

THE WORK SAMPLING OBSERVATION RECORD

In order to gather the work sampling observations in a systematic and consistent manner, a work sampling observation record is developed (Exhibit 11–4). The observation form includes a section of identifying information, e.g., department, job title, incumbent, analyst's name, date of study, and number of pages. Observation times, which vary for each day, are listed.

Time is allotted for worker preparation of the work station and for clean up. Personal time refers to coffee break, lunch break, and similar permissible time away from the work station. Even when an employee is not designated as a person to answer the telephone, this activity is included as a possible category. The worker under observation occasionally is not at the work station when the manager/analyst makes the sampling observation; this is so noted. Should excessive entries occur in this category, the manager pursues this information in detail at another time. The remaining header entries are custom-made to suit the job activities. Those given in Exhibit 11–4 reflect work of a clerical nature.

Occasionally, the analyst fails to make the observation at the time indicated. Since the number of observations missed affects the study and its reliability, it is important to include spaces where missed observations can be noted. Finally, there is room for comment, spaces to make additional notes or entries that explain and augment the observations made during the sample study. The manager develops a specific observation record for the study; prepares

Exhibit 11-4 Work Sampling Observation Record

DEPARTMENT: Medical Records

JOB TITLE: Chart Assembly

INCUMBENT: A.L. Spark

DATE:

OBSERVER: M.S. Brown

PAGE 1 OF 1

OBSERVATION TIME	Set up	Clean up	Personal	Telephone	Away from work station	Assembling charts	Checking disc. list	Pulling new folders	Obtaining Pt. ID for misc. reports	Making out control cards	Working with review Clerk	Observation time missed	Comments
9:02													
9:57													
10:18													
11:22													
12:08													
12:31													
1:16													
2:31													
3:02													
3:58													

sufficient copies of the form; chooses the observation times, either on a daily basis, or in one concentrated effort, and proceeds with the study over the designated days and weeks.

TABULATION OF RESULTS

The results obtained from the sampling study are compiled in a summary tabulation. The manager gives additional attention to areas where the results are not consistent with the expected range. Such selected areas are studied separately and in further detail, with corrective action taken as indicated. Table 11–1 shows the results of observations made of a discharge analysis clerk in the medical records division of a hospital.

CONCLUDING EXAMPLE

A final example is presented here, drawing from the direct patient care interaction. The background problem for this work sample stems from delay in patient transport from a hospital in-patient unit to the physical therapy department. The manager assesses the situation by means of the sampling technique.

Table 11–1 Example of Work Sampling Summary

Task or function	Percentage of time spent
1. Checking charts for deficiencies	36
2. Making out deficiency slips	11
3. Making out Rolodex cards	7
4. Hunting for missing charts	8
5. Assembling charts (Mondays only)	6
6. Taking charts to doctor's boxes	3
7. Away from office to pick up missing reports	2
8. Time to set up in the morning	2
9. Time to clean up desk in the evening	3
10. Filing loose reports	1
11. Personal time	20
12. Other miscellaneous duties	1
	100

Step 1. Calculate Sample Size Using Exhibit 11-1 Patient population per month = 1,000 Precision level of this study equals 4% (3.9% on the chart). This gives you a population size of 400 patients to be studied.

Summary: 400 patients needing transportation will be studied.

Step 2. Develop a Fact Gathering Form

> Time Patient Left In-patient Unit =
> Scheduled Arrival Time   =
> Actual Arrival Time   =
> Summary:

Step 3. Study Results
   a. Calculate average delay time, e.g., which inpatient unit exhibits highest frequency of delay.

Step 4. Initate Corrective Action Based on the Study.

NOTE

1. Ralph Barnes, *Work Sampling* (Dubuque: Wm. C. Brown, 1956), p. 43.

Chapter 12

Budgeting

CHAPTER OBJECTIVES

1. Identify the requisites for successful budgeting.
2. Relate budget preparation and administration to the planning and controlling function of the manager.
3. Identify traditional budget periods.
4. Identify types of budgets.
5. Differentiate between traditional budgeting and Planning-Programming-Budgeting System (PPBS).
6. Identify the steps in the budget cycle.
7. Relate the dynamics of the budget approval process to the development of the budget.
8. Identify typical budget categories.
9. Identify the steps in budget controlling through analysis of budget variances.

Budget preparation and administration are major duties of the department head. Before dealing with the actual budget calculations, the manager must understand the basic concepts and principles of budgeting. The budget details presented here are treated from the perspective of the department head rather than the accountant, comptroller, or top-level administrator. In addition, this presentation is intended for the inexperienced manager; terms are defined and examples are given in detail to facilitate budget preparation and analysis by an inexperienced user. The first part of the discussion treats basic concepts such as budget periods, types of budgets, uniform code of accounts, approaches to budgeting, and the overall budget process. The second part of the discussion focuses on the details of the budget proper: the capital expenses, personnel budget, supplies, and related expenses

Sound budgetary procedures are based on five requisites:

1. sound organizational structure so that the responsibility for budget preparation and administration is clear
2. a consistent, defined budget period
3. the development of adequate statistical data
4. a reporting system that reflects the organizational structure
5. a uniform code of accounts so that data are meaningful and consistent

USES OF THE BUDGET

Budgeting is both a planning and controlling tool. As a plan, the budget is a specific statement of the anticipated results, such as expected revenue to be earned and probable expenses to be incurred, in an operation for a future defined period. This plan is expressed in numerical terms, usually dollars. A statement of objectives in fiscal terms, the budget is a single-use plan that covers a specific period of time; it becomes the basis of future or continuing plans when the incremental approach to budgeting is used whereby the next budget is formulated through the addition of specific increments to the existing budget. It is a statement of what the organization intends to accomplish, not merely a forecast or a guess.

When the budget is properly administered, it becomes a tool of control and accountability in that it reflects the organizational structure, with each unit or department given a specific allocation of funds based on departmental goals and functions. The budget is an essential companion to the delegation of authority; the line manager who has the responsibility for developing the plans for the department or unit must be given the necessary resources to accomplish the approved plans. In turn, this manager accepts responsibility for assigning specific budget amounts to the personnel and material categories and monitoring the use of these resources. Because the budget permits a comparision of planned with actual performance, control is enhanced. The department head is responsible for those costs that are controllable, such as overtime authorization, supplies, and equipment purchases, but not for those that are arbitrarily assigned to the departmental budget, such as fringe benefits calculated as a flat percentage of personnel budget or administrative overhead calculated as a flat percentage of operating costs.

BUDGET PERIODS

A budget specifies the amount to be spent in a predetermined period. This budget period varies according to the purpose of the budget. The capital equipment or improvement budget may be developed for a long period, such as a three- or five- or ten-year period; the budget for supplies, expenses, and personnel costs may be developed for the immediate fiscal year. Given the various regulatory requirements for long-range planning and budgeting for capital improvements in health care organizations, these organizations commonly have such a combination of long- and short-term budget periods.

The usual accounting period within the overall budget framework is the fiscal year, which may or may not correspond to the calendar year. Any period equal to a full year may be chosen; this is an internal decision. Hospitals have commonly used the July to June cycle, which tends to reflect the movement of house staff at the end of the teaching year. The fiscal year may be broken into subunits of time corresponding to each of the 12 months or into 13 equal periods of 28 days each.

Periodic Moving Budget

Another approach to the definition of budget period is the periodic moving budget. In the moving budget, the basic forecast for the year is adjusted as specific periods are completed. As each period is completed, an equal time period is added:

1984	Jan.	Feb.	Mar.	
	Apr.	May	June	
	July	Aug.	Sept.	
	Oct.	Nov.	Dec.	
1985	Jan.	Feb.	Mar.	(Added when Jan.-Feb.-Mar. 1984 are completed.)

The cycle of completion and addition may be shorter, as when the July-Aug.-Sept. period is added as soon as the Jan.-Feb.-Mar. period is completed. The periodic moving budget allows the manager to make use of the more up-to-date information that becomes available as each period closes and, thus, to make a more accurate prediction.

Milestone Budgeting

In milestone budgeting, the budget periods are tied to the subsidiary plans or projects. As these milestone events are accomplished, cost can be determined and budget allocation for the next segments of the project established. The budget periods are not uniform, but depend on the projected time frame for the subsidiary plan.

TYPES OF BUDGETS

The budget may be developed to give emphasis to one of several aspects of the overall plan. The revenue and expense budget is the most common type of budget. It reflects anticipated revenues, such as those from sales, payment for services rendered, endowments, grants, and special funds, and it includes expenses, such as costs associated with personnel, capital equipment, or supplies. In the personnel or labor budget, projections are based on the number of personnel hours needed or types and kinds of skills needed rather than on wages and salaries as in the personnel costs of the revenue and expense budget. A production budget expresses the information in terms of units of production, such as economic quantities to be produced or types and capacities of machines to be utilized.

The fixed budget presumes stable conditions; it is prepared on the basis of the best information available, such as past experience and forecasting. The plans, including cost and expense calculations, are made on the basis of this expected level of activity. The variable budget concept was developed because operating costs and level of activity may fluctuate. For example, a university may calculate its unit budgets according to credit hours generated, but student enrollment may be lower than anticipated; a hospital may use dollars per patient day or average census as its basis, but the daily census in the hospital may drop and remain low. Thus, costs and expenses are established for varying rates. As actual income and operating costs become known, the budget is adjusted. The periodic moving budget is used with variable budgeting, as is the step budget.

The step budget is a form of variable budgeting in which a certain level of activity is assumed and the impact of deviations from this level of activity calculated. If the manager wishes to show several possibilities predicated on various factors, such as level of production or number of clients served, the step budget is used. These other levels may be greater or less than the basic estimate. For example, a step budget showing probable estimates plus pessimistic and optimistic allowances might be developed. The advantage of using the step budget is that it permits, even forces, the manager to examine the actions required in the event of a variation from the estimated revenue and expense. When a step budget is prepared, the fixed costs and revenues, i.e., those that are not tied to volume of service, production levels, or other factors related to operational costs, are stated. Then, the variable revenues and costs are calculated according to the volume of service, operating costs, anticipated revenues, and similar factors.

The master budget is the central, composite budget for the total organization; all the major activities of the organization are coordinated in this central budget. The department budgets are the working, detailed budgets for each unit; they are highly specific so as to permit identification of each item, as well as close coordination and monitoring of revenue and expense. In order to coordinate the several department or unit budgets into a master budget and in order to make budget processes consistent, a uniform code of accounts and specific cost centers must be developed.

The Uniform Code of Accounts

The standard classification of expenditures and other transactions made by an organization is the uniform code of accounts (also referred to as a uniform chart of accounts). Such a uniform code of accounts contains master codes and subdivisions to reflect such information as the specific transaction (e.g., personnel expense, travel, capital improvement) and the organizational unit within which the transaction occurred (e.g., purchasing department, dietary department, public relations unit). The delineation of the specific organizational unit facilitates responsibility reporting, as it is possible to relate specific expenditures to the manager in charge of that organizational unit.

The American Hospital Association, in conjunction with the American Association of Hospital Accountants, publishes a suggested code of accounts for hospitals, as well as related materials for financial management.[1] These account codes are used in the budget to group line items, such as a purchase requisition or a position authorization request. Account codes for a particular institution might include

200	Furniture
210	Capital Equipment
520	Equipment Rental
530	Equipment Maintenance and Service Contracts
580	Purchased Services (e.g., an outside contract with a coding and abstracting service)
600	Education and Travel
610	Dues and Subscriptions

Budget worksheets are coordinated with these account codes with specific items listed, line by line, under each account code. Line item is a term commonly used to refer to such specifications. For example, the worksheet for budget preparation and, subsequently, the line items of the budget for the category of Dues and Subscriptions reflect the item in detail and the unit with which it is associated.

610.1	Hospital Association dues	$ 40.00
610.2	Professional dues paid for	
	Chief of Service	120.00

610.7	Accrediting agency regulations annual update subscription	$30.00
610.8	Attendance at annual meeting of professional association	
	50% cost for Chief of Service	500.00
	25% cost for each staff assistant	250.00
	(maximum of two per year attending)	250.00
610.9	In-service Workshop for support staff (2-day seminar, in-house)	180.00

The code of accounts varies from one institution to another; the items and costs given here are for illustrative purposes only.

Cost Center

An activity or group of activities for which costs are specified, such as housekeeping, maintenance and repairs, telephone service, and similar functions, is a cost center. Usually predetermined, cost centers generally parallel the department or service structure of the organization. For example, direct patient care cost centers, with their associated codes, may include

45   Physical Therapy
46   Occupational Therapy
47   Home Care Program
48   Social Services
49   Radiology

Administrative cost centers may include

50   Data Processing and Information Service
51   Health Records Service
51   Admissions Unit
53   Dietary
54   Laundry and Housekeeping

Additional cost centers reflect costs associated with overall expense of operation:

1   Employee Health and Welfare Benefits
2   Depreciation: buildings and fixtures
3   Depreciation: equipment
4   Payroll Processing

Responsibility Center

A unit of the organization headed by an individual who has authority over and who accepts responsibility for the unit is a responsibility center. These centers parallel the organizational structure as outlined in the organization chart. The departments or services are responsibility centers, each with its detailed budget. The cost center codes and responsibility centers normally parallel one another.

APPROACHES TO BUDGETING

The two major approaches to the budgeting process are incremental budgeting and the Planning-Programming-Budgeting System (PPBS). In incremental budgeting, the financial data base of the past is increased by some given percentage. For example, the personnel portion of the budget may be increased by a flat 5 percent over the last budget period allotment, capital expenses by 7 percent, and supplies by 4 percent. There is an efficiency in this approach, since the projected calculations are relatively straightforward. There is also a danger, however; significant change, shifting priorities, or pressing need within some unit of the organization may be overlooked. As with incremental decision making, there is an implicit assumption that the original money and resource allocation was appropriately calculated and distributed among organizational units. Incremental budgets are object-oriented, i.e., they are developed in terms of personnel, materials, maintenance, and supplies. Traditional budgeting is control-oriented, while PPBS is planning-oriented.

PPBS was mandated in the Department of Defense in the early 1960s by Secretary Robert McNamara. PPBS, as the name implies, emphasizes the budgeting process in systems terms. The outputs for specific programs are assessed, and resource allocation and funding are related directly to the program goals. It is also referred to as "zero based" budgeting because past dollar allocations are not the basis of projection.

A major feature of PPBS is its departure from the traditional one-year budget cycle. Funding is projected for the period of time (frequently three or more years) needed to achieve the goals of the program. In the planning phase, the general objectives are stated and refined, the projected schedule of activities is established, and the outputs are specified. These refined objectives are grouped into programs, resulting in a hierarchy within the plans.

The alternate means of achieving the plans are assessed through cost-effectiveness analysis. Units of measure for the outputs are developed, e.g., number of clients to be served, length of hospital stay, geographical area to be covered. Cost and resulting benefit for each approach are calculated, and the best alternative in terms of cost-benefit is selected. In the PPBS approach, managers seek to increase the number of factors that can be used to provide top-level decision makers with sufficient information to make the final resource allocation. An adequate information system is, therefore, required; this is consistent with the classic systems approach, which includes an information feedback cycle.

The PPBS approach has several disadvantages. First, it is a time-consuming process, involving long-range planning, the development and comparison of alternatives in terms of cost-effectiveness, and the final budgeting. Second, not all goals can be stated precisely; not all worthy objectives can be quantified in specific measures, with a specific dollar cost attached. Third, there is the presumption that all alternatives are known and attainable. A fourth factor goes beyond the immediate dollar allocation of outright budgeting; in PPBS, the value, the legitimacy, and the actual survival of the program or organization is questioned. This, in turn, reopens conflict and exposes the accumulation of internal and external politics, the power plays, the bargaining, the trade-offs that have developed over time. The concern for program survival may intensify to the point that line managers may seek to withhold negative information and the feedback cycle may become distorted.

THE BUDGETARY PROCESS

Initial Preparation

The budgetary process is a cyclic one; the feedback obtained during one budget period becomes the basis of budget development for the next period. The budget process usually begins with the setting of overall limits by top management. The specific guidelines for budget preparation reflect the mandatory federal, state, and accrediting requirements, as well as union contract provisions and the financial assets of the organization. The timetable and particular forms to be used in budget preparation are issued along with these guidelines.

Development of the unit budget is the specific responsibility of the department manager. In some instances, a department manager may wish to use the "grass roots" approach to budgeting; unit managers or supervisors prepare their budgets and submit them to the department manager for coordination into the overall department budget. These supervisors or unit managers must, of course, be given sufficient information and guidance to carry out this function. An alternate way of involving supervisors and subordinates is to ask for suggestions about equipment needs, special resources, or supplies. In highly normative organizations, such as a university, there may be an advisory or review committee composed of selected employees who make recommendations to line officials about budget allocation. In any event, the department head bears the responsibility for final preparation, justification, and control of the budget.

The Review and Approval Process

Competition, bargaining, and compromise in the allocation of scarce resources (personnel, money, and space) occur in the review and approval phase of the budget process. It is important for the manager to have the necessary facts to support budget requests; control records to demonstrate fluctuations in the workload, staffing needs, equipment usage, and goal attainment are essential sources of such information.

The internal approval process begins with a review of the department's budget by the department head's immediate budget officer. Compliance with guidelines is checked; justification for the request for exceptions is reviewed. The organization's designated financial officer (usually the comptroller) may assist the chief executive officer in coordinating the department budgets into the master budget for the organization, but the chief executive officer is the final arbiter of resource allocation in many instances.

In the present political climate, there is increasing insistence on cost containment, and a cost containment committee may be involved in the budget review process. Current efforts for voluntary cost containment contribute to the routinization of this aspect of budget review. Cost containment committees vary in structure and mandate, but their tasks typically include advising, investigating, and even participating in the implementation of cost containment measures. Such a committee should have the questioning attitude as its primary philosophical stance; data are scrutinized and compared in an effort to identify areas where cost can be contained.

The final approval for the total budget is given by the governing board. In practice, a subcommittee on budget works with the chief executive officer, and final, formal approval is then given by the full governing board, as mandated in the organizational bylaws and/or charter of incorporation.

The budgets of organizations that receive some or all of their funds from state or federal sources may be subject to an external approval process, for example, by the state legislature or the federal Bureau of the Budget. There is a certain predictable drama in the budget process, which becomes more evident in the external review process. There is a tacit rule that budgets are padded, because budget requests are likely to be cut. The manager attempts to achieve a modicum of flexibility in budget maneuvering through overaim. There is also a necessary aspect of accountability, however. The public more or less demands that federal or state officials take proper care of the public purse. Even as clients (the public) seek greater services, they want cost containment, especially through tax relief. Public officials, then, must in fact dramatize their concern for cost containment, partly by a highly specific review of budget requests and a refusal to approve a budget as submitted.

On the other hand, should an agency request a budget allocation that is the same as, or less than, that of a previous year, serious question might be raised that the agency is doing its job. At best, the manager must recognize the subtle and overt political maneuvers that touch the budget process.

Implementation Phase

The final phase of budgeting is the implementation stage, when the approved budget allocation is spent. During this phase, revenues and expenses are regularly compared, e.g., through periodic budget reconciliation. Should revenues fall short of the anticipated amount or should unexpected expenses arise, there may be a budget freeze or certain items may be cut. For example, overtime may be prohibited; personnel vacancies may not be filled, except for emergency situations; supplies or travel money may be eliminated.

There are specific internal procedures that must be followed to activate budgeted funds in the normal course of business. For example, the budget may contain an appropriation for certain supplies, but a companion requisition system must be used to effect the actual purchase of such supplies. When an individual worker is to be hired, a position authorization request may be used to activate that position as approved in the budget. Finally, during the budget year, preparation for the following budget period is made, bringing the manager full circle in the budget process (Exhibit 12–1).

CAPITAL EXPENSES

An organization owns and operates capital facilities of a permanent or semipermanent nature, such as land, buildings, machinery, and equipment. Capital budget items are those revenues and costs related to the capital facilities. These expenses may be centralized as a single administrative cost for the entire organization, or they may be specified for each budgetary unit. The manager at the departmental level is normally concerned primarily with capital improvements for the department, such as acquisition of additional space, renovation and repairs, special electrical wiring, and painting.

Exhibit 12–1 Annual Budget Plan—Based on Fiscal Year: July 1 to June 30

Activity	Current Year												Projected Year							
	Jul	Aug	Sept	Oct	Nov	Dec	Jan	Feb	Mar	Apr	May	June	July	Aug	Sept	Oct	Nov	Dec	Jan	Feb
1. Current budget executed; monthly reconciliation & adjustments made	↑————————————————————————→																			
2. CEO & Controller develop forecasts; issue budget guidelines to departments						▮	▮													
3. Dept. Heads formulate budgets and submit								▮												
4. CEO & Controller develop master budget									▮											
5. Departmental revisions made & submitted									▮											
6. CEO & Controller finalize budget										▮										
7. Board of Trustee subcommittee review: further adjustments made and final approval given										▮	▮	▮								
8. TRANSITION: close out current year accounts												▨								
9. New Fiscal Year budget in effect OR Tentative budget in effect, pending full approval and/or further revisions													↑			↑				↑

The second capital expense in the departmental budget is major equipment. The equipment budget usually includes fixed equipment that is not subject to removal or transfer and that has a relatively long life. Major equipment that is movable is also included. The distinction between major and minor equipment is usually made on the basis of the cost and life expectancy of the item; major equipment commonly includes any item over $100.00 that has a life expectancy of more than five years. As with other aspects of budgeting, however, a specific organization may use some other cost or life expectancy factor to define major equipment/capital equipment expense. Major, fixed equipment includes the heating fixtures, built-in cabinets or shelves, and appliances; major, movable equipment includes file cabinets, patient beds, typewriters, and oxygen tents.

When budgeting for major equipment expenses, the manager may calculate acquisition cost and prorate this cost over the expected life of the equipment. Depreciation costs are a factor in equipment selection. In *Chart of Accounts,*[2] the American Hospital Association included a reference table for estimating the useful life of major equipment and a formula to calculate composite depreciation rates for each unit of equipment. An item that is more costly to acquire may be less expensive in the long run because of a lower operating cost, long life expectancy, or slower rate of depreciation. This information should be included on the supplemental information forms used to justify equipment selection.

The worksheet for capital expenses includes the account code number from the uniform code of accounts, item description, unit cost, quantity, and total cost (Exhibits 12–2 and 12–3).

SUPPLIES AND OTHER EXPENSES

The many consumable items that are needed for the day-to-day work of the department are listed under the category of supplies. It may be tempting at first to group all these items under a "Miscellaneous" category, but the clear

---

Exhibit 12–2 Sample Worksheet for Capital Expenses—Medical Records

Department: Medical Records Fiscal Year: July 1, 1984–June 30, 1985				
Account Code	Account Title: Item Description	Quantity	Item Cost	Total
210.6	Secretarial Desk	1	$485.00	$485.00
210.7	Side Chairs	3	75.00	225.00

Exhibit 12–3 Sample Worksheet for Capital Expenses—Physical Therapy

Department: Physical Therapy Fiscal Year: July 1, 1984–June 30, 1985				
Account Code	Account Title: Item Description	Quantity	Item Cost	Total
210.3	Parallel Bars - 10 foot	1	$1,025.00	$1,025.00
210.4	Shoulder Wheel - Deluxe Heavy Duty	1	225.00	225.00

delineation and listing of such items in the appropriate budget category alerts the manager to the magnitude of these costs and facilitates control. Items considered consumable supplies typically include routine items, such as pens, pencils, notepads, letterhead stationery, staples, scissors, rubber bands, paper clips. Postage is included in this category unless it is absorbed as a central administrative line item.

A given department may have special consumable supplies that are essential to its operation. The direct patient care units incur expenses related to medical and surgical supplies. The clinical laboratory has a major expense in reagents. A medical record department has as a major expense the color-coded, preprinted folders used for patient records. Special forms approved and mandated for medical record documentation (e.g., the face sheet/identification sheet used in the admission unit, the preoperative anesthesia report form used in the surgical unit, the laboratory requisition/report form for laboratory studies) may be charged to each department as they are requisitioned and used. An alternative practice is to charge the medical record department or central forms design unit with the cost of all preprinted forms. When the emphasis in the budgeting process is on control, however, it is preferable to charge the unit using such supplies so that administrative control may be fixed.

Special expenses commonly incurred at the department level include the lease and rental of equipment, the purchase of technical reference books and periodicals, training and education costs, travel and meeting expenses. Contractual services for a special activity (such as transcription, microfilming, statistical abstracting, special laboratory studies) are included under the expense category.

The work sheet for budget requests for consumable supplies and expenses typically includes the required account number from the organization's uniform code of accounts, the item description, item cost, and total requested (Exhibits 12–4 and 12–5).

Exhibit 12–4 Sample Worksheet for Supplies and Other
Expenses—Medical Records

Account Code	Account Title: Item Description	Quantity	Item Cost	Total
Department: Medical Records Fiscal Year: July 1, 1984–June 30, 1985				
610.2	Annual Professional Dues paid for Department Head	—	$120.00	$120.00
610.7	Accrediting Agency Regulations Annual Update subscription	1	30.00	30.00
610.4	Drug Usage Manual, current edition	4	7.00	28.00

Exhibit 12–5 Sample Worksheet for Supplies and Expenses—Physical
Therapy

Account Code	Account Title Item Description	Quantity	Item Cost	Total
Department: Physical Therapy Fiscal Year: July 1, 1984–June 30, 1985				
322.2	Ultrasound Gel - (gallons)	2	$13.50	$27.00
322.3	T.E.N.S. Pads - (dispensers)	10	9.50	95.00
600.4	Four Day Education Seminar		100./day	400.00

THE PERSONNEL BUDGET

Typically, personnel is the largest category of expense, accounting for as much as 85 percent of the total budget in many cases. Personnel costs include the wage and salary calculation for each position and for each worker, including anticipated raises (e.g., cost of living increases, merit increases) or adjustments resulting from a change in status (e.g., from probationary employee to full-time, permanent employee). The department manager normally calculates these costs; special justification for an increase in the number of positions or for adjustments to individual salaries or wages is also included.

Also calculated and justified by the department manager are those costs associated with vacation relief, overtime pay, and temporary or seasonal help. Specific support information may be required for these budget requests, such as a calculation of the personnel hours required to give proper departmental coverage and a calculation of the hours not available to the organization because of vacation time and holidays. If there is a high employee turnover rate or a distinct pattern of absenteeism, historical information, such as the average time lost over the past year or several years as a result of these circumstances, may be cited as support information.

In calculating the costs for personnel needs, the manager deals with impersonal costs, i.e., those associated with the position, regardless of the incumbent; such costs include the wage or salary range for the position and the number of full-time equivalent positions. In addition, there are other costs that are associated with the incumbent and change with the holder of the position; these costs include the number of hours scheduled for work each week, the number of years in the job category, eligibility for merit increases, and anniversary date for a scheduled increase in pay. The following factors must be considered in any budget calculation:

1. minimum wage. Federal law mandates a base pay rate for certain jobs. Some categories of temporary help may be exempt from this wage; the manager must seek the guidance of the personnel specialist for details of this provision.
2. union contract stipulations. Each class of job and each incumbent must be reviewed in light of contractual mandates for basic wage as well as mandatory increases. Where there is more than one contract in effect, the provisions of each contract must be reviewed and applied as appropriate. Wage and salary increases on a straight percentage basis may be mandated. In some cases, the contract may state that either a given percentage or a flat dollar amount, whichever gives the greater increase, is to be awarded. A hiring rate may be indicated for employees on "new-hire" status; a related job rate may be indicated with the employee moving to job rate at the end of the probationary period (Table 12–1).
3. organizational wage and salary scale. Except for the specific provisions of union contracts, the organizational wage and salary scale applies. Positions are listed by job category or class, and the individual employee's rate is calculated from this scale. Increases may be in terms of a percentage or in terms of step increases dependent on the number of years in the position.
4. cost of living increase. The organizational guidelines and/or contract provisions establish cost of living increases. Frequently, this amount is given as a flat percentage increase added to the base rate of pay, although it may be given as a flat dollar amount added to the base rate of pay.
5. merit raise or bonus pay. These costs may be shown as an overall amount given to the department as a whole. The manager may not be able to assign dollar amounts to an individual worker at the beginning

Table 12-1 Sample Salary Structure

Pay Grade	Hiring Rate (Weekly)	Job Rate (90 calendar days)
B	$198	$212
C	$201	$218
D	$213	$230

of a year, since the merit award may not be given until some time period has passed and the worker has earned the increase. Specific guidelines are given to the manager concerning the calculation of merit or bonus pay as part of the base rate of pay or as a one-time increase that does not become part of the employee's base rate of pay.

6. special adjustments. From time to time, a special adjustment may be made to the wage or salary structure. An organization that is adjusting its wage and salary structure to satisfy Equal Employment Opportunity Commission (EEOC) mandates may grant a one-time adjustment to a class of workers or an individual (e.g., women and/or minority workers) to bring their rate of pay in line with other workers' pay scales. When long-term employees' rates of pay "shrink" as compared with those of incoming workers, a special, one-time adjustment may be made to keep the comparative wages of new versus long-term employees equitable.

The budget worksheet and/or budget display sheet (Exhibit 12–6) generally includes the following items, which progress logically from the factual information based on the present salary of the incumbents to the projected salary through the coming budget period:

1. position code or grade code, obtained from the master position code sheet for the department and organization.
2. position description: abbreviated job title or category.
3. budgeted full-time equivalents (FTEs): the number of personnel hours per position, divided by the hours per full-time work week. Example (based on a 40-hour work week):

Worker A	40 hours
Worker B	27 hours
Worker C	20 hours
Worker D	13 hours
	100 = 2.5 FTEs

4. employee number, usually assigned by personnel division or payroll division for identification of payroll costs and employee records.

Exhibit 12-6 Personnel Budget: Medical Record Department, Fiscal Year

Grade Code	Position Title	PT/FT Day Eve	Incumbent	Current Bi-Weekly	Projected Annual Base	Anniv. Date	Projected Annual Increase	Projected Total Salary	Hours Per Pay Period Bi-Weekly
3	Coding/Abstr. clerk	FT-D	P. Hart	304.00	7,904	8/6/83	280.00	8,184	80
3	Record Locator clerk	FT-N	H. Reinhold	304.00	7,904	12/8/83	203.00	8,107	80
4	Release of Info. clerk	FT-D	T. Maloney	336.00	8,736	3/17/84	92.00	8,828	80
5	Quality Assurance								
	Assistant	FT-D	M. Caretto	400.00	10,400	5/31/84	34.00	10,434	80

5. employee name: name of incumbent. If position is vacant, this information is noted.
6. actual FTEs: number of employed workers and number of vacancies.
7. current rate of pay: hourly rate, biweekly rate, or job rate. The hourly rate is calculated by dividing the total salary by the number of work hours per budget period; the biweekly rate, by dividing the total salary by 26. The job rate is usually specified in the wage scale, especially as given in a union contract.
8. projected annual base salary, calculated by multiplying the rate by the appropriate unit of time. This projected salary is specific to the incumbent. Should the incumbent separate from the organization with the replacement worker hired at entry-level pay, the annual base salary would be lower.
9. incumbent's anniversary date, used to calculate cost of living or other raise associated with date of employment.
10. projected annual increase because of cost of living increase, merit or bonus pay, or special adjustments.
11. projected total salary: present salary plus projected annual increase.

DIRECT AND INDIRECT EXPENSES

A department budget also reflects costs under the categories of direct and indirect expenses. Direct expenses typically include salaries, services and contracts, dues and subscriptions, and equipment. Indirect expenses are charged to the departmental budget on a formula basis or some process of assessment. These indirect costs are associated with the organization as a whole and are prorated per department. Examples of indirect costs and their units of assessment are shown in Table 12–2.

Table 12–2 Indirect Expenses Charged to Medical Record Service

Item	Amount	Basis of Calculation
Fringe benefits/health and welfare	$70,000	% of salaries
Equipment depreciation	8,200	Depreciation schedule
Telephone costs (equipment)	5,484	Number of telephones
Maintenance and repairs	2,000	Number of work orders
Physical plant operation (e.g., heat, air conditioning)	42,000	Number of square feet
Building depreciation	6,000	Number of square feet

BUDGET JUSTIFICATION

As mentioned earlier, support or explanatory documentation may be required for budget requests. If a particular type of equipment is requested, the manager is expected to explain why that particular model or brand is needed. Reasons may be compatibility with existing equipment, guaranteed service contracts, availability, or durability. Projected patient usage is another element of support data; the acquisition of a particular item may enhance patient care because of its safety features, or it may attract more patients to the facility. Sometimes an item may be needed simply to remain competitive and thereby retain a given patient population. The budget justification may take the form of a cost comparison, such as that between rental/long-term lease of equipment and outright purchase plus maintenance costs. For a medical record department, the cost comparison of in-house word processing/transcription unit and contractual service might be included.

Development of Fee Schedule

In direct patient care services, the details of the fee schedule may be part of the budget support information. The income generated on the basis of the fee schedule must, at the least, meet expenses. Profit-making institutions must determine their profit base and add this percentage to the established fee schedule. The criteria employed in developing a fee schedule that accurately compensates a department for the services it renders is used as part of the budget justification.

The following discussion illustrates the development of a fee schedule for a physical therapy department. Many physical therapy departments have established fee schedules primarily on the basis of supply and demand, existing fee schedules in other departments in the community or surrounding area, actual time involved in administering a treatment, the number of modalities used, and cost of equipment. In order to establish an equitable fee schedule, many of these factors should be considered. Before this can be done, however, it is necessary to determine the total costs of a physical therapy service.

Rodriquez and Rodriquez developed a cost accounting method that provides a formula to determine costs for physical therapy services.[3] This method involves separating the services into three components:

1. direct labor costs, including physical therapists' salaries and all fringe benefits
2. equipment costs, including the original purchase price or ongoing leasing costs of the equipment, depreciation schedule, maintenance and repair costs

3. overhead costs, including nonprofessional labor costs, telephone, rent, utilities, cleaning and maintenance, and all the other expenses of operating the program

The Rodriquez and Rodriquez formula is based on a cost per hour for each of these three components.

Formula for Determining Value of Treatment*

Computing Hourly Labor Cost

1. Add the total number of hours worked per month by all the therapists to determine monthly pay hours.
2. Take 70% to 80% of monthly pay hours to determine monthly production hours.
3. Divide monthly production hours into your monthly therapist's salary to determine your average productive hourly rate. This is the hourly cost.

Computing Hourly Equipment Cost

1. Divide the initial cost of equipment by the estimated number of years of expected life.
2. Add 10% of the initial cost for maintenance and repair.
3. Add 6% of the initial cost for interest on investment. *Note:* Because the information is based on 1955 estimates, the inflation % should be increased accordingly.
4. Assume the equipment will be used 20% of the potential hours of use.
5. Divide the sum for the first three items by #4. This gives you the hourly equipment cost.

Computing Hourly Overhead Rate

1. Take 45% plus or minus of the maximum patients or treatment rooms per hour. This represents patients per space per hour.

---

*Reprinted from *Physical Therapy* (35:298, 1955) with permission of the American Physical Therapy Association.

2. Apply hours or the equivalent days per week times 4.3
weeks per month. This will determine the patient space
hours per month.
3. Divide the average monthly overhead expenses by the patient space hours per month to determine the average
hourly overhead rates.

The rates obtained when using this formula may be applied to
determine the actual cost of a prescribed treatment session.

Modifications of the Rodriquez and Rodriquez formula on establishing a
schedule of charges for physical therapy services have been outlined in the
literature.[4,5,6] Certain factors have a profound effect on this formula, such as
the number of hours available for administering patient treatments, the
number and type of patients being treated, and the size of the department,
including the number and type of staff employed and their productivity.

Time Unit System

Another method of establishing a fee for services is a time unit system
developed by Jagger and May.[7]* Their approach is based on the total cost of
providing the service for a specific length of time. Patients pay for services
according to the amount of time they spend in the department each day.

Before the fee schedule is established as proposed by Jagger and May, the
cost of operating the total program, both direct and indirect cost, must be
calculated. Direct costs usually include salaries, fringe benefits, therapeutic
supplies, educational travel, and other expenses over which the Director of
Physical Therapy has control. Indirect costs usually include charges to the
department for services provided by the institution, such as utilities, mail and
telephone services, housekeeping and general maintenance, as well as the
cost of housing the department. Indirect costs are assigned in many ways,
but they are generally computed on the basis of square footage. The hospital
accountant or financial officer can assist the department head in gathering
this information.

Once the total cost of operating the department has been established, the
units of time available to recover that cost through charges to the patient
must be determined. Regardless of how many hours per week a department
is open, charges can be assessed only on the actual time the therapist has
available for patient care. Therapists must also devote some time to support

*Adapted from *Physical Therapy* (56: 536–540, 1976) with permission of the American
Physical Therapy Association.

activities, such as attending clinics or rounds, writing notes in the medical record, and meeting with other health care professionals. In addition, therapists provide nondirect patient care, such as supervising patients who may be practicing a skill on their own.

A study conducted at the Eugene Talmadge Memorial Hospital of the Medical College of Georgia revealed that therapists whose major responsibilities were in providing patient services devoted 60 percent of their time to direct patient care activities, 10 percent to nondirect patient care, and 30 percent to support activities.[8] Each facility must determine the percentages of available direct and nondirect time. These figures vary among general hospitals, medical center teaching facilities, and outpatient services.

The number of hours the percentages of direct and nondirect time represent for each therapist must be determined. On the basis of a 40-hour week, each therapist is theoretically available 2,080 maximum hours each year. However, vacation time, sick leave, attendance at educational seminars, and other similar activities reduce the total available hours per year. The maximum and actual number of hours available per therapist for patient care is computed as follows:

1. maximum number of hours available per therapist per year; weekend coverage not included (52 weeks × 40 hours per week = 2,080).
2. actual available weeks per therapist per year (52 weeks minus 2 weeks vacation, 1 week sick leave, 1 week educational leave = 48).
3. actual available hours per therapist per year (48 weeks × 40 hours per week = 1,920).
4. hours available for direct patient services per therapist (1,920 hours × 60% time spent in direct patient service = 1,152).
5. hours available for nondirect patient services (1,920 hours × 10% time spent in nondirect services = 192).

After determining personnel time available for direct and nondirect patient care, the manager calculates total FTEs for all personnel involved in the delivery of patient services, i.e., full-time and part-time physical therapists and physical therapy assistants. Since the primary role of the physical therapy aides is to provide support services, they are excluded in determining available time units.

The number of time units per hour to be used as the base for the time unit system of fee setting is arbitrary. This unit of time can be 5 minutes, 10 minutes, 20 minutes, or any number of minutes as determined by the department. Most hospitals use 15 minutes as the basic time unit. If 15 minutes is used as the base time unit and there is a professional staff of physical therapists and physical therapy assistants of 6.5 FTEs, the total time units available for patient care is determined by multiplying the total available hours by 4.

1. total time units available for direct patient care (1,152 hours × 6.5 FTE × 4 = 29,952).
2. total time units available for nondirect patient care (192 hours × 6.5 FTE × 4 = 4,784).
3. total available time units (29,952 + 4,784 = 34,944).

In many institutions, especially rehabilitation facilities, patients spend additional time practicing activities initially taught by the physical therapists. For example, the physical therapist may be involved with the patient for one hour on a one-to-one basis, and the patient may use the facility for two additional hours to practice activities. Since the patient is using the facility for direct instruction and for practice, it is proper to establish two fees: (1) a personnel time unit fee to cover the cost of all personnel involved in direct care, and (2) a facility time unit fee to cover the time spent in the department during direct and nondirect care time.

To establish the personnel time unit fee charge, the cost of the professional staff (FTEs) involved in providing direct patient care, including their portion of the fringe benefits, is subtracted from the total operating budget of the department (direct and indirect expenses). Next, the cost of professional staff (FTEs) providing direct patient care is divided by the number of time units available for direct patient care, thereby establishing the personnel time unit fee.

$$\frac{\text{Professional staff costs (FTEs) + fringe benefits}}{\text{Time units for direct care}} = \frac{\text{personnel time}}{\text{unit fee}}$$

The facility time use fee is computed by dividing the adjusted cost of operating the department (minus the costs of the professional staff and their fringe benefits) by the total available time units.

$$\frac{\text{Adjusted operating cost of the department}}{\text{Total direct} + \text{Total nondirect}} = \frac{\text{Facility}}{\text{time unit}}$$
$$\text{time units} \quad \text{time units} \qquad \text{fee}$$

The charges to a patient can be seen in the following example. An amputee spends a total of three hours a day in the department: one hour of direct care and two additional hours practicing activities on his own, but still under the supervision of the physical therapy department staff. Using the 15-minute base as the time unit, the patient is charged for the following:

Personnel fee: 4 units
Facility fee: 12 units

The charges determined under the time unit system reflect the patient's use of resources in terms of time, supplies, and a share of the indirect costs.

BUDGET VARIANCES

During the fiscal year, the manager receives periodic reports showing budgeted amounts versus amounts spent. This report may categorize such information under the headings of "over budget" or "under budget" for the period and for the year. The manager uses this information as a monitoring and control device. A particular unit's budget may include money for overtime that is assigned arbitrarily to budget quarters. A periodic report may show that the manager was over budget in that category for the quarter, but not for the year. Such a report is an internal warning system that alerts the manager to that line item. Filed with higher level management, the variance report reflects the manager's awareness of the expenditure for the quarter and its relationship to the yearly amount as a whole. Should there be some unexpected cause for utilizing these overtime funds, such as high absenteeism because of employee illness or injury, this information is noted in the variance report.

Under budget indicators require similar explanations as part of the control process in budgeting. Explanations for under budget items are not required in every instance, but particular attention must be given to large sums that have not been spent because of delay factors in the outside environment. For example, the purchase of a large, expensive piece of equipment may be included in the budget for the fiscal year. If it is not available until the next fiscal year, the delay could throw a carefully planned budget out of balance; i.e., funds are not expended in one year, and no funds are allotted for this purchase in the upcoming budget. The manager should anticipate such a situation and make arrangements for the transfer of funds in a timely way.

Direct patient care service budgets include projections of care to be rendered. Actual revenue generated per patient visit is compared with projected revenue. The explanations—over or under projections of care to be rendered—are made by the budget officer for the service. If patient care services are below those projected, plans for increasing services may be included with the explanation.

NOTES

1. American Hospital Association, *Chart of Accounts* (Chicago: American Hospital Association, 1973).

2. Ibid.

3. Arthur A. Rodriquez and Alfred Rodriquez, "A Schedule of Charges for Physical Therapy Services," *Physical Therapy* 35, no. 6 (June 1955): 295–298.

4. James McKillip, "Criteria for Establishing Fee Schedules," *Physical Therapy* 42, no. 5 (May 1962): 303–306.

5. James W. Price, "Setting Rates for Physical Therapy Services," *Physical Therapy* 49, no. 3 (March 1969): 265–268.

6. Robert Hickok, ed., *Physical Therapy Administration and Management* (Baltimore: Williams & Wilkins, 1974), pp. 91–114.

7. Dilys M. Jagger and Bella T. May, "Time Unit System of Fee Setting," *Physical Therapy* 56, no. 5 (May 1976): 536–540.

8. Ibid., p. 538.

Chapter 13

Management by Objectives

CHAPTER OBJECTIVES

1. Define management by objectives (MBO).
2. Identify the advantages of MBO.
3. Relate the concept of participative management to MBO.
4. Relate motivational theory to MBO.
5. Identify the participants in the MBO process.
6. Identify the MBO cycle.
7. Identify the characteristics of performance objectives in MBO.
8. Relate MBO to operational goals.

Management by objectives (MBO) or results management is a process of planning, motivating, and controlling in which the resources of the organization are focused on achieving the key objectives stated in the organization's overall goals. MBO provides a framework within which the personnel and the resources of the organization are assessed continually in the light of specific goal attainment. The overall goals are emphasized, the impact of the work of a unit or division on total organizational effort is recognized, and the decisions to allocate organizational resources are made in a manner that optimizes overall performance. MBO is an integrative management concept, containing elements of the planning process, participative management, motivation, and control. It reflects the systems approach to management with its emphasis on a cycle of planning, effecting, and feedback with assessment of change in the input-output cycle.

HISTORICAL DEVELOPMENT

Several parallel events in management history led to the development of MBO. These events include the work of behavioral scientists, who stressed the value of motivation and participation, and the application of MBO concepts to business and industrial long-range planning. Table 13–1 contains selected concepts in the development of MBO within the last two decades.

The manager in contemporary health care organizations should understand the MBO concept, since its use in health care management is increasing. A hospital, for example, may use this approach for its administrative reports, as well as in its budget process. MBO may be required for research or special project grants; for example, the Department of Health, Education and Welfare (HEW) required MBO as the management process for developing the programs funded under its 1974 grants for trauma research.

Table 13–1 History of Management by Objectives

Date	Originator/Source	Key Concept, Term, or Point of Emphasis
1954	Peter Drucker *The Practice of Management*[1]	Introduction of the term *management by objectives*
1960	Douglas McGregor *The Human Side of Enterprise*[2]	Theory X and Theory Y of motivation; value of self-direction and self-control in working toward objectives
1961	Rensis Likert *New Patterns of Management*[3]	Behavioral science applied to management theory; emphasis on self-set goals and related self-set controls as more effective than imposed goals and controls
1965	George S. Ordiorne *Management by Objectives*[4]	Development of extensive written materials on MBO
1967	John Humble *Management by Objectives in Action*[5]	Development of detailed material for application of MBO
1960s		Long-range planning with adoption of MBO process in business and industry

ADVANTAGES OF MBO

Major reasons that have been identified for using MBO include the following:

- Rational organizational planning is more readily achieved; long-range plans become actualized through highly coordinated derived goals.
- Communication is facilitated through the management conference process; upward and downward communication flows in a systematic manner.
- Performance is monitored as an aspect of control; results of specific plans are examined in the performance review conferences, during which individual performance is assessed.
- Motivation is enhanced because of routine involvement of key participants.
- The authority-responsibility patterns are reinforced where the work to achieve the goal is performed; this clarity of authority and responsibility adds to both the motivational and the control aspects of the process.
- Training needs are identified and anticipated; the opportunity for individual development is provided.

MBO is adaptable to the budget process, as specific objectives can be linked to requests for allocation of money and personnel. Demonstrating objectives planned and objectives accomplished within a time frame corresponding to the budget cycle provides the manager with comparatively strong budget justification. MBO may be linked to Planning-Programming-Budgeting System process in this way.

The budget justification sometimes takes the form of management by objectives. The manager is required to relate budgeted costs to objectives to be achieved. The objectives for this documentation are similar (even exact wording) to the objectives of the department. Progressive accomplishment throughout the year would be charted through traditional MBO statements. For example, see Exhibit 13-1.

Another use of MBO is in concert with the PERT network (see Chapter 10). As the activities needed to complete the many network events are delineated, the MBO components of objectives, target date, and responsibility are readily identified.

RELATIONSHIP TO PARTICIPATIVE MANAGEMENT

MBO emphasizes participative management, i.e., the involvement of each individual affected, as far as practicable, in the planning process, decision making, and assessment of results. Not only are the skills and abilities of

Exhibit 13-1 Sample MBO Statement

Departmental Objective: (ongoing objective)
  Provision of all records requested for clinic use

  Intermediate objectives:
  a. increase staffing in file area for morning shift.
     Estimated hours per week: 24
     Projected cost per week: $182.00

     Time frame: July through September

  b. Prevent backlog in file area during vacation season
     Estimated hours per week: 65
     Projected staffing:
             overtime for 25 hours = $100.00
             temporary help for 40 hours = $220.00
     Time frame: July through September

  c. Conversion to new work shifts in October to provide coverage from 7:00 A.M.
     through 8:00 P.M.

     Shifts to be seven hours each with some overlap to meet peak demands for clinic
     requests.

     Eliminate temporary help and overtime.

---

these individuals assessed, but also the planning and decision-making process is opened so that they may become emotionally and mentally involved. It is more than involvement at skill level; it is involvement of the self.

The purpose of participative management is to motivate the individuals to work toward the goals; it also helps elicit critical information from the supervisory and line workers. It enhances the acceptance of change, since the individuals affected by the change understand the reasons for it more fully. Participative management also encourages workers to accept responsibility for the activities, because they view the success of the plan as their own success; they help to determine the areas of responsibility rather than have responsibility imposed on them. The participative leadership style is the presumed authority relationship in the MBO process.

UNDERLYING MOTIVATIONAL ASSUMPTIONS

MBO may be linked with certain behavioral science assumptions about worker motivation. Self-motivation is stressed. Theory Y as described by Douglas McGregor reflects the management view of worker motivation that is consistent with MBO.[6] Basic tenets of the behavioral school of thought on motivation include

• Employees want to know what is expected of them.

• Employees want to participate in and influence decisions affecting their performance.

• Employees want feedback on how they are performing.

• Employees' performance is affected positively by supervisor interest in their work.

PARTICIPANTS IN MBO

Who participates in MBO? Does MBO mean that the manager sits down with each and every employee? Do workers plan the details of the work within some overall boundary set by the manager? Is this a realistic approach to work? One could raise the objection: what manager has that kind of time? How can my workers make management decisions? The level of MBO participation that is desirable varies; there is no absolute number of key participants. In some discussions of MBO, there is an implicit inclusion of all workers at all times. In others, the emphasis is on management pairs or small management-worker teams. The degree of participation and the point of participation in the MBO cycle depends on several factors.

The basic participants are, first of all, the management pair. A manager, at any level of the organization, and the manager's immediate assistant or supervisor constitute the first level of participants in the MBO process. These individual officeholders have the fundamental charge to develop goals and policies consistent with overall organizational goals and to carry them out. The concept of management pairs may easily be broadened to include other managers and supervisors who are concerned with the same derived objectives and the same workflow, and who hold successive levels of authority and responsibility in the chain of command for a department. A review of the organization chart rapidly reveals potential key participants. Successive groups of supervisors or workers become involved as the plans are developed within each department or unit.

A health care organization may have an explicit goal of providing continuity of care. This goal invests all the departments with a fundamental charge to carry out activities to support continuity of care. An assistant administrator in charge of several departments, such as the admission unit, the medical record service, and patient information service, may call together the managers of these three departments to develop specific objectives for their departments to support continuity of care. Each of these managers in turn carries the MBO process into his or her department and develops the appropriate operational objectives with the supervisor or assistant director involved with activities that are central to this goal. In this pattern of participation, the MBO planning and feedback process is limited to those with clear management roles. The process may be carried another step by having these second- and third-level assistants and supervisors use the specific MBO cycle in their planning. It is at this level that immediate line workers become involved.

Factors that must be taken into account to determine the appropriate degree of worker involvement include the nature of the work, the degree of training of the workers, and the time frame imposed for achieving the goals. Many of the same factors that determine the appropriate span of management (see Chapter 5) may be significant in determining the appropriate level of worker participation as well. Participation is restricted to those areas of work in which the worker has the knowledge and training to make a meaningful contribution.

MBO CYCLE

There are three distinct phases in the MBO cycle: the planning phase, the performance review phase, and the feedback phase leading to a new planning phase. Table 13–2 summarizes the MBO cycle in terms of each phase, key activities for the phase, and the participants involved in each phase. To illustrate these phases, Table 13–3 presents an example of the MBO cycle as followed in an occupational therapy program.

Planning

The overall organizational goals are identified and stated. If this has been done in a prior planning phase, these goals are reaffirmed at the start of the MBO cycle. As noted earlier, many goals are recurring ones, such as maintaining accreditation of a hospital or an educational program, serving a distinct client group, or developing outreach programs. Specific departmental objectives are agreed upon within the framework of the overall objectives.

Selection of objectives is the basic activity on which the MBO process is built, and it must be given careful attention. A guiding principle for the choice of objectives is the rule of the critical few, also referred to as the

Table 13–2 Summary of MBO Cycle

Phase	Key Activities	Participants
Planning	Identifies and defines key organizational goals	Manager
	Identifies and defines key departmental goals that stem from overall goals	
	Identifies and defines performance measures (operational goals) for employees	
	Formulates and proposes goals for specific job	Subordinate
	Formulates and proposes measures for specific job	
	Participate in management conferences	Manager and subordinates
	Achieve joint agreement on individual objectives and individual performance	
	Set up timetable for periodic meetings for performance review	
Performance review	Continue to participate in periodic management conferences	Manager and subordinates
	Adjust and refine objectives based on feedback, new constraints, and new inputs	
	Eliminate inappropriate goals	
	Readjust timetable as needed	
	Maintain ongoing comparison of proposed timetable and actual performance through use of control monitoring devices, such as visible control charts	
Feedback to new planning stage	Reviews overall organizational and departmental goals for the next planning period, such as the next fiscal year	Manager

Table 13-3 Example of MBO Cycle

Date: 9/17
Project: Reorganize program by December 31.

Phase	Key Activities	Participants
Planning	Review present program by 9/22	Director
	Prepare goals for patient dressing, bathing, and toileting activities by diagnostic categories by 9/30	Alice M., staff therapist
	Prepare goals for patient dressing, bathing, and toileting activities by patient functional ability by 9/30	Lenny R., staff therapist
	Compare goal statements and amended goals by 10/5	Director and staff
	Hold conference to discuss goals	Director and staff
	Formulate draft goals by 10/12 and circulate among staff	Director
	Final amendment of goals by 10/15	Director
Performance review	Introduce new program to patients; adjust goals and report during supervisory meetings	Director and staff
	Hold staff meetings every Friday for two months	Director and staff
Feedback	Confer with other department heads and supervisors regarding quality of new program by 11/15	Director
	Refine activities of daily living program as per suggestions and feedback; circulate among staff by 11/15	Director
	Meet with patients and families to assess progress in individual cases and summarize findings by 11/15	Staff

Pareto principle. In essence, this concept reflects the probability that most of the key results will be generated by only a few of the activities, while most of the activities will generate only a few of the key results. Pareto estimated that the relationship was 20 percent to 80 percent in most situations; that is, 80 percent of the results would be derived from 20 percent of the objectives, while 80 percent of the objectives would generate only 20 percent of the key results. Priority of effort, then, may be given to those objectives identified as "the critical few."

The following examples illustrate the characteristics of properly formulated objectives. Quantifiers and the deadlines, as well as the designation of responsibility, are included.

- File clerk to complete audit of files to detect and correct misfiles in sections 00-38-76 to 00-99-76 by October 26.

- Director of Medical Record Department to recruit an assistant director specializing in medical care evaluation; to be done by December 15, for starting salary of not more than $15,200.

- Transcription unit supervisor to reduce backlog of discharge summaries by 50 percent by November 1. Reduce error rate per operative report by 10 percent by December 15.

The following examples, which correspond to those listed above, would be incorrect because they are too vague; they lack either a quantifying or qualifying element and there is no assigned deadline or responsibility.

Example 1: Reduce misfiles in permanent storage area.
Example 2: Hire an assistant to help with additional workload in medical record department.
Example 3: Reduce backlog and eliminate all typing errors in transcription unit.

Just as the statement of objectives must be realistic, the time frame for the accomplishment of objectives must be realistic. The time frame must be long enough to permit achievement of the objectives yet short enough to permit timely feedback and intervention. Through careful estimates of such factors as required training time, seasonal changes in workflow, or the availability of personnel or supplies, or budgetary considerations, a timetable can be developed that leads to accomplishment of the objectives.

A natural time frame is given when MBO is linked to the annual budget period. This questioning process requires managers to rejustify the existence of the programs. Another easily identifiable time frame stems from deadlines imposed by outside agencies, such as a one-year provisional accreditation or the two-year full accreditation by the Joint Commission on Accreditation of Hospitals (JCAH). If MBO is linked to a special project that is planned and controlled through a PERT network, the time frame coincides with the overall project target date, and the target dates for the completion of each set of activities correspond to events in the network. Within the overall time frame, management conferences are scheduled to assess progress and to adjust plans.

Performance Objectives

In the MBO process, the performance objectives developed are essentially operational goals or objectives. The objectives that are determined for an MBO sequence should be distinguished by three characteristics:

1. specificity. Each objective should include a plan that shows the work to be done, the time frame within which it is to be accomplished, and a clear designation of the individual who is to accomplish the work.
2. measurability. Each objective, as far as possible, should have quantitative indicators for the measurement of work accomplished. If an activity cannot be quantified, qualitative factors should be developed.
3. attainability. Each objective should be realistic; it should be possible to carry out the activity within the time frame established.

Performance objectives have much in common with operational goals, which will be discussed here briefly, in conjunction with their use in management by objectives.

Operational Goals

In addition to the formal statements of objectives and desired functional statements of performance, a manager may wish to develop operational, or working, goals for internal department use only. Operational goals are also highly specific, measurable, and attainable; they must be sufficiently concrete to relate the overall goals and objectives to specific action. When the statement of objectives and the related functional objectives are sufficiently refined and stable, there may be no need for operational goals.

Operational goals may be seen as temporary measures that take into account the reality of changing, usually difficult, work situations. They reflect the impact of a high turnover rate, absenteeism, employees in a trainee status, physical renovation of the work area, or temporary emergency situations. Operational goals may become progressively more refined as progress is achieved in certain areas. In a training program, for example, the operational goals may be relatively lenient with respect to error tolerance or the time required for accomplishment of the work. As the trainee progresses to full employee status, the work standards and related operational goals become stricter, moving gradually toward the desired formal objectives. In MBO, when a situation is problematical, the performance objectives may have the flavor of operational goals; a plan is made to move, by specific target dates, from the present situation to the desired goal. Thus, the time frame, the amount of work to be accomplished, and similar factors, are stated in a realistic fashion, always in concert with the final goal—full compliance or full satisfaction of departmental goals.

Performance Review

The performance objectives determined in the MBO conference must be fair, based on all known relevant conditions, adjusted to the individual's capability, and adjusted to the specific constraints of the work situation. The objectives themselves do not vary from one performance meeting to another, but the points to be measured are subject to change because of variations in conditions during work cycles. The worker may be involved in special training and, therefore, may be given a more modest output to attain at the beginning; later, the quantity or the quality may be set at a higher level. At another phase in the work cycle, some new constraint may be identified, such as equipment problems, unanticipated turnover in workers, or an unexpected surge in client demand; a consequent adjustment in quantity may be made.

The purpose of performance review is not only to monitor the performance, but also to make adjustments as indicated by the situation. Successful use of MBO includes the allowance for a margin of error, i.e., planning for mistakes and accepting the human factor. This planning for contingencies gives realism to the objectives and is helpful in enhancing employee acceptance of the process.

Feedback

There are several, even many, management conferences to formulate the original plans, to adjust these plans during the performance review phase, and to obtain the necessary feedback. During the management conferences between workers and managers, specific planning takes place:

1. Appropriate objectives are identified through mutual agreement.
2. Time periods for achieving the objectives are established.
3. Responsibility in terms of results is defined.
4. Revision and adjustments are made periodically.

The feedback process is structured and includes a review of the specific control documents that were developed to monitor progress, such as visible control charts, PERT network activity specification sheets, and training plans. Reasons for failure to meet objectives are documented; these factual data are assessed and plans adjusted accordingly. The purpose of the interim feedback is to facilitate corrective action. There should be no punitive element to the conferences.

In addition to the periodic review of the work, an overall review is done at the end of the cycle, with the identification of objectives, constraints, and time frame for the next cycle.

FORMATS FOR MBO PLAN

The format for writing a detailed MBO plan varies; managers develop a format to suit their own needs unless a specific format is imposed by a higher authority in the organization. Exhibits 13–2 through 13–5 illustrate the essential components and relationships of the MBO plan. Regardless of what format is used, certain information should be included routinely in the MBO plan:

- department
- unit or subdivision
- overall objectives and the derived operational objectives
- the period covered in the MBO cycle
- key participants
- workflow factors and special constraints
- identification of training needs
- methods of evaluation to be used
- detailed time plan

Exhibit 13–2 MBO Plan: Example 1

Department	Medical Record Department
Unit/subdivision	Transcription unit
Overall objective	To develop and maintain a system of dictation and transcription for the timely and accurate processing of medical record entries.
Derived operational goals/specific objectives	To transcribe all priority reports within four hours of receipt. To transcribe all other reports within 24 hours of receipt.
Key participants	1. Director, Medical Record Department 2. Assistant Director 3. Transcription Unit Supervisor

Exhibit 13-2 continued

Workflow factors	1. Assistant Director to check on problems stemming from delays in receipt of transcription belts from outpatient clinic area; to be done during June. 2. Transcription Unit Supervisor to have all equipment serviced by June; no new equipment budgeted for coming year.
Anticipated constraints	1. Vacancy anticipated owing to one employee's maternity leave August through January. 2. Vacation time mid-June through September. 3. Surge of transcription as residents change services and/or leave at end of June. 4. Uncertainty concerning budget; not usually approved until two to three months into budget cycle; uncertain allotment of money for overtime or additional temporary help, at least from July through September. 5. Close out of budget; use all available money from this budget for overtime or temporary help during late June.
Workers involved	See organization chart; all transcriptionists and Unit Supervisor; Assistant Director to give overall explanation of program; Unit Supervisor to work with each transcriptionist to identify special needs. Target date: first week in June.
Training needs	1. Only one worker trained to use automatic typewriter; train second worker. 2. All have completed basic terminology course, but need specialized terminology. 3. Assistant Director to develop 16-hour medical terminology course; to be given in two stages—June and September.
Methods and standards for control	Continue to use present work standard of 800 lines per day, error-free; monitor overall unit output through visible control chart.
Detailed time plan	Meeting dates: April 17 May 8 May 15 June 4

Exhibit 13–3 MBO Plan: Example 2

Department: Occupational Therapy
Unit: Rehabilitation

Overall Objective:

1. To offer quality occupational therapy to patients in the clinic and in the patient's room.

Derived Goals:

1. Pick up referrals within 24 hours.
2. Evaluate patients and report to physician within 72 hours of receipt of referral.
3. Treat all patients daily.
4. Participate in family and team conferences.
5. Teach home programs to family members.
6. Plan for patient's discharge.

Key Participants: Director of OT; OT staff and secretary

Workflow Factors:

1. Director to log all references and check on evaluation schedule.
2. Director to develop ADL schedule on ward.
3. Secretary to time/date all referrals.
4. Secretary to notify staff of pending discharges.

Anticipated Constraints:

1. Referrals may back up in physicians' offices.
2. Staff given short notice of discharges.
3. Family conferences scheduled during treatment times.
4. Secretary planning to resign next month.
5. Budget constraints force therapists to treat minimum of four patients per hour.

Workers Involved:

Director; 3 staff occupational therapists (OTR); 3 occupational therapy assistants (COTA); 1 secretary

Training Needs:

1. Therapists must keep skills current.
2. Therapists must attend continuing education programs.

Methods and Standards for Control:

1. Therapists must evaluate 2 patients per day.
2. Therapists must treat 8 patients.
3. Ongoing quality assurance program as detailed for hospital.

Exhibit 13–4 MBO Plan: Example 3—Yearly Cycle of Consultant
Activity in Long-Term Care Facility

	Focus	Medical Record System	Chart Content
Jan. Feb. Mar.	Admissions	1. Patient care policies 2. Procedures: chart development at time of admission 3. In-house filing 4. In-service: patients' rights and consents	1. Patients' rights form 2. Consent forms 3. Face sheet completion 4. Admission physical 5. Initial progress note 6. Initial physician notes 7. Initial physician orders 8. Nurse's notes on admission
Apr. May June	Transfers	1. Transfer agreement 2. Patient care policies re transfers 3. Release of information 4. Exchange of information at time of transfers	1. Transfer orders 2. Completion of transfer form 3. Documentation: receiving a patient as a transfer; sending a patient as a transfer
July Aug. Sept.	Medical Documentation	1. Patient care policies re medical documentation 2. Chart review procedure; emphasis on in-house review 3. Adequacy of chart review list	1. Physician orders 2. Progress notes 3. Histories and physicals: at admission, annual
Oct. Nov. Dec.	Discharges	1. Processing charts at discharge 2. Coding and indexing 3. Statistical compilations 4. Permanent files	1. Discharge orders 2. Discharge summary 3. Final nurse's notes 4. Diagnoses 5. Death certificate

Exhibit 13–5 MBO Plan: Example 4

Department	Physical Therapy
Unit	Spinal Cord Unit
Overall Objective	To develop an educational handbook of patient care for respirator-dependent quadriplegics.
Derived Goals	To teach patients, families, and hospital personnel the care and progress of the respirator-dependent patient.
	To standardize information presented by the professional staff on the care of the patient throughout the period of hospitalization.
	To provide a quick reference for individuals involved in posthospitalization care of the respirator-dependent patient.
	To complete the handbook by May 4.
	To present completed handbook to Spinal Cord Unit Executive Committee on May 18.
Key Participants	Physicians
	Nurses
	Physical Therapists
	Occupational Therapists
	Speech Therapists
	Psychologists
	Social Workers
	Project Coordinator
Workflow Factors	1. Physicians to chair committee and also to provide medical information.
	2. Members of other disciplines to provide written procedures on the care and progress of the patient, including any equipment needed.
	3. Committee members to critique information presented by the various disciplines for clarity and understanding.
	4. Project coordinator to compose information presented at each meeting and prepare draft copy of the handbook.
	5. Final draft of the handbook to be presented to the Spinal Cord Unit Executive Committee for approval prior to printing.

Exhibit 13–5 continued

Anticipated Constraints	1. Limited time available for committee personnel to be involved in the project. 2. Committee members absent from meetings. 3. Committee member not meeting established timetable. 4. Lack of adequate support staff for typing and collating information. 5. Lack of sufficient funds to print completed handbook.
Workers Involved	Physicians Representatives of each discipline involved in the care of the respirator-dependent quadriplegic patient.
Training Needs	1. Member of each discipline involved in the care of the respirator-dependent quadriplegic patient will be responsible for educating respective staff personnel about the written procedures contained in the handbook. 2. The social worker will be responsible for the distribution of the handbook to current patients in the Spinal Cord Unit and to newly admitted patients.
Methods and Standards for Control	1. Prior to discharge, the handbook to be reviewed by member of each discipline treating the patient to ensure all pertinent information has been included. 2. Follow-up questionnaire to be sent to each patient six months after discharge. 3. Questionnaire to be returned to the Project Coordinator for summarization prior to presentation to the respirator-dependent patient handbook committee.

Detailed Time Plan	Meeting dates
	   January 5
	   February 2
	   March 2
	   April 6

NOTES

1. Peter F. Drucker, *The Practice of Management* (New York: Harper & Row, 1954).
2. Douglas McGregor, *The Human Side of Enterprise* (New York: McGraw-Hill, 1960).
3. Rensis Likert, *New Patterns of Management* (New York: McGraw-Hill, 1961).
4. George S. Ordiorne, *Management by Objectives* (New York: Putnam, 1965).
5. John W. Humble, *Management by Objectives in Action* (New York: McGraw-Hill, 1970).
6. McGregor, *The Human Side of Enterprise.*

Part II

Organizational Environment and Dynamics: The Context of Management Practice

Chapter 14

The Organization as a Total System

CHAPTER OBJECTIVES

1. Understand the uniqueness of an organization by assessing the organizational environment.
2. Differentiate between an informal organization and a formal organization.
3. Classify organizations according to primary characteristics.
4. Classify health care organizations according to various organizational types.
5. Identify the characteristics of classic bureaucracy.
6. Identify the consequences to the manager of the organizational environment.

Social evidence abounds with support for the basic observation that man forms groups: the family, the clan, the neighborhood, the church, the political party, a business, a fraternity, a work group, a professional association. The study of these groups as social organizations is the proper domain of the social scientist; their study as formal organizations is the proper focus of administrative analysis.

The successful manager recognizes the impact of the organizational environment on clients, members of the organization, and the public at large, as well as on the manager's specific role. An organization does not exist in a static world; rather, it is in a continual state of transaction with its environment. As an open system, the organization receives inputs from its environment, acts on them and is acted on by them, and produces outputs, such as goods, services, and even organizational survival as an essential, primary output. Consequently, the organizational environment consists of both internal and external components. The specific functions of the manager are modified by the organizational environment, i.e., the specific attributes of a given work setting. Classic organizational theory provides the manager with concepts to assess the organizational environment.

The organizational environment may be assessed by an examination of its characteristics and components through a typology of organizations, a review of the organizational life cycle, and an analysis of its purpose and functions. The use of clientele network and systems models yields further information about the internal and external components of the organizational environment. Managers may anticipate organizational conflict when stated purposes or goals and actual practices become disparate; such an occurrence should alert managers to changes in the organizational environment so that they can develop an anticipatory response rather than a reactive response.

FORMAL VS. INFORMAL ORGANIZATIONS

An organization is a basic social unit that has been established for the purpose of achieving a goal. A formal organization is characterized by several distinct features:

1. a common goal, an accepted pattern of purpose
2. a set of shared values or common beliefs, giving individuals a sense of identification and belonging
3. continuity of interaction that is goal-oriented
4. a division of labor and specialization, deliberately planned to achieve the goal
5. a system of authority or a chain of command to achieve conscious integration of the group and conscious coordination of effort to reach the goal

An informal organization may be characterized by some of the features of the formal organization, but it lacks one or more of these features. Individuals who share a common value may meet regularly to foster some goal, and this group may become a recognizable formal organization. Some informal groups never develop the consistent characteristics of a formal organization, however, and simply remain informal.

Formal organizations almost inevitably give rise to informal organizations. Such informal groups may be viewed as spontaneous organizations that emerge because individuals are brought together by the common workplace, common goal, and inescapable social interaction. Informal organizations arise as a means of easing the restrictions of formal structures, as in the cooperative communication and coordination that may occur outside of the officially mandated channels of authority. Through the informal organization's communication network, an individual may gain valuable information that supplements or clarifies the formal communications. Through the informal grouping, individuals are integrated into the organization and are socialized to accept the specific organizational role assigned to them. A manager must remain aware of the existence and composition of the informal groups in the organization so that their functioning affects the formal structure in positive rather than negative ways.

CLASSIFICATION OF ORGANIZATIONS

When an organization's managers understand and accept its nature, organizational conflict can be reduced and organizational viability increased, because the managers function in a manner consistent with the type of organization shaping the interactions. Personal conflict can be reduced. Should an individual be unwilling or unable to accept certain aspects of a particular organizational type, that individual may decide to move to a different organizational climate. For example, if an individual practitioner prefers not to function in a highly structured, bureaucratic setting, it is better to recognize this before accepting employment in a government-sponsored health care institution. An individual who believes that health care should not be "for profit" would do well to seek employment in health care settings that are not predicated on the business model. An individual may gain an insight into the climate of a particular organization through the use of organizational classifications, such as prime beneficiary, authority structure, and genotypic characteristics.

Prime Beneficiary

Peter Blau and W.R. Scott presented a classification of organizations in terms of prime beneficiary.[1] Their suggested model for the analysis of organizations has as its basis the question: Who benefits from the existence of the organization? Four types of organizations result from the application of this criterion:

1. mutual benefit associations where the membership is the prime beneficiary; examples include a professional association, a credit union, and a collective bargaining unit
2. business concerns where the owners are the prime beneficiaries
3. service organizations where the client group is the prime beneficiary

4. commonweal organizations where the public-at-large is the prime beneficiary, such as the military or fire department[2]

Managers may formulate goals, establish priorities, and monitor activities
to determine the effectiveness of the organization in meeting the needs of the
prime beneficiary. Actions that do not foster such goals are eliminated and
proper priorities formulated. Because the clients are the prime beneficiaries
of a service organization, decisions about hours of service, scope of service
offered, and similar matters are made with the needs of clients in mind. In
health care, the growing development of home care, flexible hours in outpatient care clinics, and alternatives to full hospitalization are attempts at
meeting the needs of the prime beneficiaries, the patients and their families.
At the same time, collective bargaining among health care worker units
represents the mutual benefit association. Managers in health care settings
must balance the demands made by both types of organizational forms within one organization.

Authority Structure

The organizational environment can also be classified according to the
modes of authority that are operative in the institution. Managers must
adopt leadership styles, develop procedures and methods for worker interaction, and determine client interactions in a manner that is consistent with the
predominant authority structure. Health care organizations tend to embody
more than one pattern of authority structure; for example, there are few
limits on the activities of professional staff and greater limits on the semi-
skilled and unskilled workers. The work of Amatai Etzioni provides a typology of organizations based on the authority structure predominant in the
institution.[3] The classification that results from this approach may be summarized as

1. predominantly coercive authority: prisons, concentration camps, custo-
dial mental institutions, or coercive unions
2. predominantly utilitarian, rational-legal authority, use of economic rewards: businesses, industry, unions, and the military in peacetime
3. predominantly normative authority; use of membership, status, intrin-
sic values: religious organizations, universities, professional associations, mutual benefit associations, fraternal and philanthropic
associations
4. mixed structures: normative-coercive, e.g., combat units; utilitarian-
normative, e.g., most labor unions; utilitarian-coercive, e.g., some early
industries, some farms, company towns, ships

Genotypic Characteristics

Like the prime beneficiary concept, the classification of organizations by genotype is based on an analysis of their fundamental roots and purposes. Daniel Katz and Robert Kahn viewed organizations as subsystems of the larger society that carry out basic functions of that larger society. These basic functions are the focal point in this system of classification. The typology of organizations developed by Katz and Kahn is based on genotypes, or first order characteristics: What is the most basic function that the organization carries out in terms of society?[4] These first order, basic functions are as follows:

1. productive or economic functions: the creation of wealth or goods, as in businesses
2. maintenance of society: concern with the socialization and general care of people, as in education, training, indoctrination, restoration of health
3. adaptive functions: the creation of knowledge, as in universities, research, artistic endeavors
4. managerial/political functions: adjudication and coordination functions, control of resources and people, as in court systems, police, political parties, interest groups, government agencies

The charter, articles of incorporation, and statement of purpose are official documents of the organization that can be used to classify the organization according to this typology.

Goal statements are derived and priorities set in terms of primary function. Managers can monitor organizational change when the actual function performed differs from the stated function. When a social service agency spends a great deal of effort determining eligibility of patients for service under a variety of government programs, it is assuming some of the characteristics of a managerial/political organization. Sometimes this adjudication interferes with the delivery of the health care service; managers must make decisions in the light of this conflict. If priority is given to research and education over direct patient care, the health care practitioner must again come to terms with the true nature of the organization.

CLASSIFICATION OF HEALTH CARE ORGANIZATIONS

When the health care organization is classified according to these typologies, the complexity of the setting becomes apparent. Classification by prime beneficiary offers several possibilities. In terms of direct patient care, for example, the health care organization can be classified as a typical service organization. On the other hand, if it is a for-profit institution, classification as a business organization is more appropriate. If the health care organization has a mixed goal, as does a teaching hospital associated with a medical school, it can be defined as a service organization with its clients—both the physicians to be educated and the patients to be treated—the beneficiaries. The potentially conflicting priorities of teaching and direct patient care underlie the selection of patients for treatment, however; preference may be given to those patients who are "interesting" case material for teaching purposes. Even when a health care institution is not directly associated with a medical school, a variety of clinical affiliation arrangements may be developed to meet the needs of such practitioners as occupational and physical therapists, medical technologists, social workers, health records administrators, dietitians, and other groups that require clinical practice as part of their educational sequence. In developing goal statements for a department, the chief of service must keep this secondary goal in mind.

The health care organization also is a commonweal organization insofar as it protects the public interest in matters of general community health, such as the benefits of the facility's research efforts to the public at large. Health care institutions also offer a variety of free health-monitoring programs as a means of fostering health maintenance in the community at large.

Etzioni included the hospital as an example of normative authority structure. This point could be argued, however, depending on the focus of organizational analysis. Professional staff members tend to function in the normative mode; their codes of ethics, professional training, and the general level of behavior expected of them modify individual participation in the organization as much, if not more, than do formal bylaws and contractual arrangements. In this sense, the normative authority structure predominates. When the health care organization is viewed from another perspective, it seems to function more as a mixed normative-utilitarian structure. With business orientation and the increasing unionization of workers in the health care field, the utilitarian model seems to be a more appropriate category.

A coercive element is sometimes introduced into the health care setting, as when individuals are assigned to health care jobs in wartime as an alternative to military service or when hospital volunteer work is given as part of a court sentence. This makes the health care institution involved a mix of normative-utilitarian-coercive authority and requires the manager to adopt a variety of leadership and motivational styles in working with these different groups in the organization. Worker/member motivation and the source of the manager's authority differ for these different groups involved with the organization.

In the Katz and Kahn genotypic classification, the health care organization fits two categories, again indicating the mixed mandates of such entities.

As an organization concerned with restoration, the health care establishment functions to maintain society. It also performs adaptive functions when higher education (e.g., medical school) and research are major goals.

CLASSIC BUREAUCRACY

Bureaucracy is such a common aspect of organizational life that it is often treated as synonymous with formal organization. The study of bureaucracy in its pure form was the work of the structuralists in management history: Max Weber, Peter Blau and W. Richard Scott, and Robert K. Merton. Weber's work is pivotal since it presented the chief characteristics of bureaucracy in its pure form. Weber regarded the bureaucratic form as an ideal type and described the theoretically perfect organization.[5] In effect, he codified the major characteristics of formal organizations in which rational decision making and administrative efficiency are maximized. He did not include the dysfunctional aspects or the aberrations that occur when any characteristics are exaggerated, as in the popular equation of bureaucracy with "red tape." From the works of Weber and others,[6] a composite set of characteristics or descriptive statements may be derived concerning the formal organization or bureaucracy:

1. size
   a. large scale of operations, number of clients, volume of work, and geographical dispersion
   b. communication beyond face-to-face, personal interaction
2. division of labor
   a. systematic division of labor
   b. clear limits and boundaries of work units
3. specialization
   a. a result of division of labor
   b. each unit's pursuit of its goal without conflict because of clear boundaries
   c. areas of specialization and division of labor that correspond with official jurisdictional areas
   d. specific sphere of competence for each incumbent
   e. promotion of staff expertise
   f. technical qualifications for officeholders
4. official jurisdictional areas
   a. fixed by rules, laws, or administrative regulation
   b. official duties specific for each office

5. rational-legal authority
   a. formal authority attached to the official position or office
   b. authority delegated in a stable way
   c. clear rules delineating the use of authority
   d. depersonalization of office; emphasis on the position, not the person
6. principle of hierarchy
   a. firmly ordered system of supervision and subordination
   b. each lower office or position under the control and supervision of a higher one
   c. systematic checking and reinforcing of compliance
7. rules
   a. providing continuity of operations
   b. promoting stability, regardless of changing personnel
   c. routinizing the work
   d. generating "red tape"
8. impersonality
   a. impersonal orientation by officials
   b. emphasis on the rules and regulations
   c. disregard of personal considerations in clients and employees
   d. rational judgments, free of personal feeling
   e. social distance among successive levels of the hierarchy
   f. social distance from clients
9. the bureaucrat
   a. career with system of promotion to reward loyalty and service
   b. special training required because of specialization, division of labor, or technical rules
   c. separation of manager from owner
   d. compensation by salaries, not dependent on direct payment by clients
10. the bureau (or office or administrative unit)
    a. formulation and recording of all administrative acts, decisions, and rules
    b. enhancement of systematic interpretation of norms and enforcement of rules
    c. written documents, equipment, and support staff employed to maintain records
    d. office management based on expert, specialized training
    e. physical property, equipment, and supplies clearly separate from personal belongings and domicile of the officeholder

These characteristics are interwoven, one flowing from the other; for example, the growing size necessitates a division of labor, which, in turn, fosters specialization.

One of the dreams of many direct patient care practitioners is a health care delivery system that does not become bogged down in formalities. The private practice model seems to offer the solution; if the private practice or small group practice flourishes, however, the characteristics of formal organizations inevitably begin to emerge, e.g., specialization and division of labor procedures for uniformity, some form of authority structure, and a variety of rules. The wisest approach seems to involve taking the best features of formal bureaucracy and making particular efforts to avoid the negative elements, such as impersonality. Family-centered approaches to health care or the team approach are models that tend to offset the impersonalization associated with large health care organizations.

CONSEQUENCES OF ORGANIZATIONAL FORM

Managers work in specific organizational environments, and their specific functions are shaped and modified by the organizational form, structure, and authority climate. Some specific consequences of organizational form and climate include

- size. The more layers in the hierarchy, the greater (potentially) the limits on managers' freedom in decision making. Their decisions may be subject to review at several levels, and more decisions may be imposed from these higher levels.
- organizational climate. The degree to which clients, workers, and other managers participate in planning and decision-making processes is determined in part by the authority climate. Managers may have to modify their management/leadership style if it is inconsistent with the organization's authority structure. The basis of motivation may vary. In the highly normative setting, for example, members willingly participate; in the coercive organization, the basis of motivation tends to rest on the avoidance of punishment.
- the degree of bureaucracy in form. A highly bureaucratic organization may be associated with great predictability in routine practices, but less innovation and more resistance to change. The effort to offset distortion caused by layering in communication may be a predominant activity for the manager in a highly bureaucratic organization.
- the phase in the life cycle. The openness to innovation and the vigorous, aggressive undertakings through goal expansion and multiplication that

characterize some stages of the life cycle may permit the manager to undertake a variety of activities that are precluded by concerns for organizational survival in other phases of the life cycle.

For these reasons, managers must assess the organizational setting and their own roles. The major concepts of the clientele network, organizational life cycle, and analysis of organizational goals are tools for such analysis. Their active use fosters in the manager an awareness of the overall organizational dynamics that shape managerial practice, worker interaction, and client service.

NOTES

1. Peter Blau and W.R. Scott, *Formal Organizations* (San Francisco: Chandler Publishing Co., 1962), p. 42.

2. Ibid., p. 43.

3. Amatai Etzioni, *A Comparative Analysis of Complex Organizations* (Glencoe, IL: The Free Press, 1961).

4. Daniel Katz and Robert L. Kahn, *The Social Psychology of Organizations* (New York: John Wiley & Sons, 1967), p. 11.

5. Max Weber, *The Theory of Social and Economic Organization,* A.M. Henderson and Talcott Parsons (trans.) and Talcott Parsons (ed.) (Glencoe, IL: The Free Press, 1947), pp. 324–386.

6. H.H. Gerth and C. Wright Mills, *The Theory of Social and Economic Organization,* trans. A.M. Henderson and Talcott Parsons, ed. Talcott Parsons (Glencoe, IL: The Free Press and Falcon's Wing Press, 1947), pp. 324–386.

Chapter 15

The Clientele Network

CHAPTER OBJECTIVES

1. Define the concept of clientele network.
2. Identify the impact on management activities of each group in the clientele network.
3. Understand the significance of support, competition, and rivalry among groups within an organization.
4. Apply the concept of the clientele network to the health care setting.

A major charge given implicitly to any manager is the building of external relationships. In order to do this, the manager must identify critical relationships, develop satisfactory working relationships with the several key individuals and groups involved, and, finally, work at maintaining these relationships. With the conservation of organizational resources, time, money, and personnel as a mandate, the manager seeks to capitalize on available external sources of power, influence, advice, and support, as well as to identify those areas of potential difficulty, such as competition and rivalry, erosion of client good will, and shifting client demand and loyalty. In an era of increasing regulation of health care, the contemporary manager in the health care setting must identify and comply with multiple sets of changing regulations and guidelines issued by federal and state government agencies as well as by the various accrediting agencies, such as the Joint Commission on Accreditation of Hospitals (JCAH) or the American Osteopathic Association.

Like a living organism, an organization has a dynamic environment to which it must continually adapt. The manager identifies these units and constructs a network of the pattern of interrelationships. Bertram Gross developed the concept of the clientele network (Figure 15–1), noting that any organization is usually surrounded by a complex array of people, units, and other organizations that interrelate with it on the basis of various roles. He called these people, units, and organizations the "publics with opinions."[1]

Wherever the concept of organization is used, a department manager could well substitute individual service or department. Although such a department or service is obviously a part of the organization, the development of the clientele network for a unit within the organization yields information about the critical relationships, clients, adversaries, and supporters of that department. Department level managers must be aware of the unique environment of their department or service, as well as the overall environment of their organization.

Figure 15–1 The Clientele Network

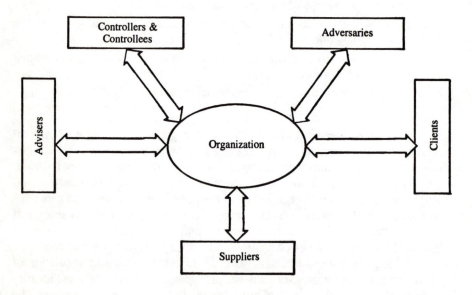

PUBLICS WITH OPINIONS

CLIENTS

The most obvious and immediate individuals and groups who make significant demands on the organization are the clients. Gross used the term in a broad sense of clients as customers, i.e., those for whom goods and services are provided by the organization.[2] Immediate, visible clients in health care, both for the organization and for any department directly involved in patient care services, are the patients.

The providers of direct health care services are immediate, visible clients for certain units within the organizations. The business office, the legal staff, and the medical record department offer support services to assist physicians, nurses, and social workers in the provision of patient care. Given the traditional and historical development of the modern hospital, it could be said that the physicians are a special class of clients in that the organization of the hospital or clinic gives them the necessary support personnel and services for patient care. Physicians within their specialties are clients to each other, depending on each other for consultative services and referrals.

Certain services may be placed into the client category vis-a-vis each other. Some services, such as physical therapy, are income-producing units; because the resources obtained are used on behalf of the whole organization, other units may be considered clients of the income-producing group. The business office relies on the medical record service to supply certain documentation to satisfy financial claims, and the safety committee relies on the several patient care and administrative departments to supply the information necessary to perform its function.

The use of the broadest possible definition of client alerts the manager to the subtle facets of organizational relationships. The manager who recognizes the number of distinct client groups can more effectively monitor their several, and sometimes, conflicting demands for services.

Although one step removed from the immediate services or goods offered by the organization, less visible clients are nonetheless legitimate users of the services or goods. By identifying these secondary clients, the manager has a key to the primary and secondary goals of the organization or unit. In the many educational programs offered within health care organizations, for example, the sponsoring institutions (e.g., a college or university), the health professionals and the technical students are secondary, less visible clients. Hospitals traditionally have direct patient care as a primary goal, with teaching and research as secondary goals. The ordering of priorities should stem from recognition of the multilevel client demands.

The same physicians who are immediate clients in terms of their need for support services for their direct patient care activities are less visible clients in terms of their need for opportunities for education and research. The employees of the organizations are a kind of less visible client, since one of the organizational outputs is the provision of jobs. Occasionally, in health care, the provision of jobs is an explicit goal; the neighborhood health centers sponsored by the federal government were intended not only to provide health care services, but also to afford job opportunities to area residents.

The clients twice removed from the immediate goal of the organization may be termed the remote clients. Many of these individuals and groups do not even know they are being served. In addition to patient care, teaching, and research, a third goal of health care organizations is generally given as the protection of the public at large, i.e., remote clients.

The manager, in assessing the stated and implied goals, may readily identify them by analyzing the needs of primary, visible clients, as well as those of the less visible and remote clients. If the client demand is relatively stable, the planning, organizing, and staffing functions of the manager may be done on the basis of some predictability; that which can be predicted can be reasonably controlled. Workflow, organizational pattern, and staffing needs may be assessed in a stable manner. The net effect is efficiency in the allocation of resources of money, space, and personnel.

There is within the client group a potential capacity to control the organization. When a business has only one major purchaser of its goods or an agency has only one group to serve, the clients could easily take charge of the organization, limiting its independence. On the other hand, the organization with multiple clients must set priorities, balance conflicting demands, and maneuver so as to satisfy several groups.

SUPPLIERS

Three categories of suppliers are given by Gross: (1) resource suppliers, (2) associates, and (3) supporters.[3]

Resource Suppliers

Since no organization is totally self-sufficient, it must take into itself the necessary resources, raw material, money, and good will that it needs to survive and function. In this sense, the organization is the client of other organizations.

Within the given organization, one department or service is the supplier of another. In assessing workflow patterns, this concept is useful in identifying which aspects of the work are within the unit's immediate control and which originate in one or several other departments. The medical record department is the client of several other units in this sense. The proper gathering of patient identification information is the work of the several admissions and intake units; a medical record department is dependent on these units for that part of the workflow. Resource suppliers, such as the ward clerk/secretary, control the medical record at the time of a patient's discharge; consequently, its timely receipt in the medical record department after discharge is somewhat dependent on that unit's workflow. A centralized, computerized data-processing system is dependent in the same way. The laboratory or radiology department, physical therapy department, and occupational therapy department all depend on the nursing service literally to bring, send, or prepare the patient so that they can proceed with their own work in a predictable manner. Essential information for the formulation of job descriptions concerning interdepartmental relationships or for the development of cross-training programs within the organization is obtained from an awareness of those organizational components that act as resource suppliers to each other.

In the same sense, the chief executive officer can be seen as a resource supplier, making the final adjudication in the allocation of space, money, and personnel to the units. The manager of the department or service should know the needs of other departments and should develop strategic alliances in the competition for scarce resources.

Associates

Individuals or groups outside the organization who work cooperatively with the organization in a joint effort are associates of the organization.[4] Associates have a common interest and common work that unites them with the organization. The manager who recognizes the efforts of associates will actively obtain their cooperation. Through informal sharing of ideas among themselves, the various health care practitioners frequently act as associates to each other. The medical record practitioners from several area hospitals may collaborate informally on a release of information policy so that there is areawide consistency in dealing with requests for data from patient records. The medical technologists of a region may cooperate in a joint venture for blood banking processes.

Supporters

Various politically, socially, and economically powerful individuals and groups in the society may be supporters of the organization. They mobilize "friendly power" for the organization, giving it encouragement and developing a climate of good will toward the organization. Such supporters can coordinate major activities, such as fund raising, public relations, and intermediate services for the organization. This type of support helps the organization to conserve its own resources for direct application to immediate goals, such as providing direct patient care. Individual organizations may quite simply lack the power to mobilize certain political or economic resources on their own behalf and may depend on a "friend in the castle" to help in these matters. The traditional pattern of appointing the political, social, and economic elite to the board of trustees in health care organizations is often an effort to mobilize such power on behalf of these organizations.

Occasionally, a nationally prominent figure demonstrates a particular interest in health care because of some personal experience with a particular health problem. In a sense, poliomyelitis, heart disease, and breast cancer received more attention because they affected a president or a member of his family. A leading political figure may work toward the passage of legislation on behalf of some specific health care need; the Kennedy interest in mental health and mental retardation was a factor in the development and passage of the Community Mental Health Act of 1964. A number of well-known entertainers and sports figures have supported fund-raising activities for one or another health care issues, e.g., the Jerry Lewis Telethon for Muscular Dystrophy. Such individuals command resources unavailable to a single institution.

The Lions Club programs to support eye care, the Easter Seal program in fund raising and coordination of volunteers to work with handicapped persons, and the Shriners' traditional support of health care for crippled children illustrate the typical activity of supporters. The traditional hospital auxiliary is yet another example of a support group. Supporters may help to coordinate activities to the mutual benefit of all participants, offsetting the destructive aspect of competition and facilitating compliance with standards set by controllers by making resources available for use by the organization.

Although an organization may not actively declare itself a supporter, the net effect of its activities may provide support. The concern of the American Civil Liberties Union for privacy in general, for example, has helped raise the social consciousness of the public toward all issues concerning privacy, thus helping health care institutions to develop guidelines for the restrictive release of information. In such situations, collaboration in development and lobbying of pertinent state legislation becomes possible.

Supporters may have something to gain by actively supporting an organization. An electric company actively distributes a booklet prepared by the Society for the Prevention of Cruelty to Animals. This booklet contains information about the proper care of dogs, including appropriate times to restrain such pets (e.g., when the electric meter must be read). The benefits from such support activity are obvious.

ADVISERS

Although they are like supporters in some ways, advisers have more specific activities that tend to set trends for the industry. Advisers provide a particular form of resource or support through their advice. Gross stressed an important difference between supporters and advisers; i.e., the assistance and support of the advisers help the organization use its resources and support from the several other sources.[5] Advisers stand apart from the organization and often have a more impersonal relationship with the organization than do supporters.

The advice may be in the form of overall guidelines, position papers, data analysis, sample procedures and methods, or model legislation. Examples of advisor activity include

- American Hospital Association, Guidelines on Patient Rights

- American Medical Association, Model Legislation Concerning Disabled Physicians

- American Medical Record Association, Position Paper on the Confidentiality of Patient Records

CONTROLLERS

Those individuals or, more often, groups who have power over the organization are controllers. Health care organizations must comply with the regulations of several federal and state government agencies, for example, as well as with the mandates of the various accrediting agencies. Table 15-1 gives a listing of organizations and agencies that have such control power over the organization. The level of detail varies greatly from the optimal standards stated by JCAH to the highly detailed regulation (e.g., required room size) in a state law.

Certain controllers are internal to the organization and yet constitute a kind of separate organization. Workers as individuals are a part of the organization, but the unions that represent them stand outside the organization, exerting specific pressure on it. The governing board is an integral part

Table 15–1 Key Controllers

Controller	Requirement
Federal government	Conditions of participation for Medicare and Medicaid, special standards resulting from specific program funding and grants
State government	Institutional licensure regulations, individual professional licensure regulations
Local government	Zoning codes, fire and safety requirements
Accreditation bodies	Accreditation standards
Professional associations	Codes of conduct, professional educational requirements
Collective bargaining agreements	Detailed contract provisions
Organizational policy	Detailed provisions for each organizational unit
Various regulatory agencies	Personnel laws and regulations, such as Civil Rights Act, Worker Compensation, Fair Labor Standards Act, Occupational Safety and Health Act
Third party payers	Detailed contractual provisions concerning patient eligibility, mode of treatment covered, and similar provisions

of the hierarchical structure, but in some ways the board of trustees is separate from the line managers, who are controlled by the decisions made by the top-level management group. The assessment of the net effect of such controllers' input gives the manager a sense of clear boundaries for planning and decision making. However innovative an idea might be, for example, the manager must still keep management practices in line with these constraints.

Controllers may also impose conflicting regulations on the institution, such as the mandate of the federal government to maintain almost absolute confidentiality of alcohol and drug abuse records and the mandate of third party payers to provide satisfactory evidence of treatment for reimbursement. Managers may be forced to change their managerial style as a result of certain constraints imposed by a controller, e.g., the details of a union contract may limit severely the use of a laissez faire style of management. By means of survey questionnaires and site visits, the manager may assess the net effect of these multiple regulations on workflow, services offered, staffing patterns mandated, and job descriptions restricted and refined.

ADVERSARIES

Health care traditionally carries overtones of great compassion and deep charitable roots. Like any other organization, however, health care organizations have opponents and enemies, as well as competitors and rivals. The rising cost of health care tends to make health care professionals and the organizations in which they work a source of conflict and even a target for opposition at the present time. Indeed, clients themselves at times take an adversary stance.

Outright opponents or enemies are those individuals or groups who seek actively and aggressively to limit the organization in its activity. These opponents or enemies may have the power to bring an activity to a halt or to prohibit an activity from being started. For example, clients do not wish to have certain facilities, such as drug treatment centers or group homes for the mentally retarded, too close to their homes. Furthermore, they may want ample parking and easy access to their hospital, but they do not want to disturb the local housing units or the business areas. Zoning codes may be enforced in order to prevent the development of alternative treatment facilities or the expansion of existing facilities. Clients may withdraw financial support as evidence of displeasure.

The concept of competition is well understood and accepted in the economic arena. Within reasonable boundaries, competition is favorable for clients because it forces providers to make products or services better and/or more available. The sharp edge of competition is also evident in health care delivery, possibly because certain factors in contemporary culture are producing shifts in client loyalty. These factors include (a) erosion of strong ethnic and religious ties to one hospital or health center; (b) the passage of the Civil Rights Act, which removed certain prejudicial barriers to access; (3) urban/suburban migration patterns; (d) lowered birth rate; (e) the passage of the National Health Care Planning and Resource Development Act, which mandated the certificate-of-need process and created the Health Systems Agencies (HSAs).

Given a dropping inpatient census, a hospital may compete actively with a free-standing medical clinic by offering its own outpatient clinic services. In order to attract patients, one obstetrics unit may offer the latest in fetal monitoring, while another may stress family-centered childbirth. An urban medical school/medical center may offer the benefits of highly specialized techniques to offset a census dropping because certain clients seek to avoid the city. A hospital seeking HSA approval for an expanded facility or for some special activity may engage in active outreach to increase its patient population.

Rivals, according to Gross, are those who produce different products, but compete for resources, assistance, and support.[6] In the health care setting, specialty hospitals could be considered the rivals of general hospitals, e.g., a children's hospital versus a pediatrics ward in a general hospital, a lying-in hospital versus an obstetrics unit. When the emphasis in definition is placed on competition for the same resources, there is evidence of rivalry among health care institutions for scarce personnel, e.g., registered nurses for the 3 P.M. to 11 P.M. shift, trained medical transcriptionists, physicians for the emergency room.

Within an organization, one department may be cast as rival to another for needed space, additional personnel, and special funds. Managers may find that the same departments that are clients may also be supporters and rivals.

Additional discussion of competition and rivalry may be found in the discussion of Bureaucratic Imperialism (Chapter 16) and in Conflict and Cooperation (Chapter 17).

CASE STUDY: EXAMPLE 1

Many individuals and groups affect the management of a single unit. The elements of the clientele network are identified in this review of the Registry of Melrose Occupational Therapists, a private practice group that includes five full-time and two part-time therapists. The organization was developed by Mary S., who is now the president of the corporation. The group members hold contracts with three home health agencies and two nursing homes. Mary S. supervises the members, who treat patients daily. The group members are paid for their work on a fee-for-service basis, meaning that they are paid for direct service only. Fringe benefits are not available, because the therapists are not employed by the agency in the traditional employer-employee relationship.

The clients are immediately recognizable as the patient population. For the Melrose group, these patients either reside in their own homes or in a nursing home. When Mary S. receives a referral, she forwards the request to the appropriate therapist, who then visits the patient, performs an evaluation, and designs a treatment regime. Physical, emotional, social, and cognitive aspects of the patient's illness must be considered during the treatment process. In some instances, the families of these patients enter the picture and become additional clients in the sense of this network analysis.

Less visible clients are the agencies that hold contracts with the group. The agencies determine the services that are required and the rate of reimbursement. They supervise the quality of the services and will take action if services are not meeting the needs of the patients. The agencies need the therapists to provide these selective services, thus creating a mutuality of interaction.

The Melrose group members use their professional knowledge and skills to promote independent living for their patients. At the same time, the members must satisfy the needs of their other clients, the home health agencies and the nursing homes that hold contracts for their services. The existence of several client groups influences the decision making and priority setting in which the manager of this group engages.

Resource suppliers offer (1) material goods, such as splinting equipment; (2) emotional support, such as a newspaper article that describes a new type of service; and (3) financial support, such as items donated to raise money for special needs. Each agency is a resource supplier because it supplies necessary administrative items, such as the charting forms for documenting patient progress, and payment for each patient treatment. Furthermore, some agencies provide the therapist with splinting supplies, adaptive equipment, and exercise modalities. Each of these items may seem somewhat inconsequential individually, but the cumulative effect of resource provision may spell economic success or failure for a private contractual group such as this small agency. Attention to such detail also reduces interorganizational misunderstanding and conflict, freeing energies to be directed at patient care.

The Melrose group also acts as a resource supplier. In one nursing home, group members order eating equipment and toileting supplies for the nursing staff, thus freeing nursing personnel for direct patient care. The therapist also constructs wheelchair and bed positioning equipment.

Susan S., a Melrose Registry member, and Barry Z., a member of the Austin Practice, are developing a check-off progress note. Barry and Susan are designing this progress note to facilitate documentation of patient progress. Therapists can check off patient services that are routine and use the space at the bottom of the progress note form to focus on new areas. The form will benefit members of both private practices. Barry Z. is an associate of the Melrose group; Susan S. serves in the same capacity for the Austin group.

The Melrose group is fortunate to have a supporter in the college of health professions at the local university. Alice D. teaches in the college's occupational therapy department. When prospective clients call to ask for community services, Alice refers the calls to this private practice group.

Advisers can be compared to supporters, but their activities are more specialized and their relationship is further removed from the organization. John G., a lawyer who drafted the state licensure bill, is an adviser to the Melrose group. This lawyer's research for the licensure bill helped to delineate clearly the roles of the physical and the occupational therapists, and the Melrose group used his services when they developed guidelines for their own practice. The activities related to the drafting of the licensure bill provided this lawyer with a sensitivity to the problems that arise in daily practice within these specialties.

Controllers are evident in the variety of contractual relationships into which the Melrose Registry must enter. The group holds contracts with the Bureau of Health Insurance, Worker Compensation Bureau, Sun Insurance Company, Blue Cross and Blue Shield, Consolidated Medical Service/Health Maintenance Organization, and the Anderson Nursing Home Association. Each of these organizations has established its own guidelines and regulations concerning reimbursement. The individuals who work for the Melrose group define their list of reimbursable services to fit the criteria of the controller; the nature of these decisions shapes the scope of the practice.

Other controllers include the American Occupational Therapy Association, the only national organization for occupational therapists. The association provides guidelines for private practice, ethics, and standards. The American Physical Therapy Association and other professional groups provide guidelines to deliver patient services.

The Melrose Registry seems to have no outright opponents and enemies, but there is the natural competition with other private practice groups. The members once concentrated on pediatric evaluation, but the interests of the group members now extend to nursing homes. Northwood Health Services, which has been in the nursing home contract service business for several years, is a competitor of the Melrose group. Adversaries need not be enemies. In health care it is advisable to work cooperatively. Members of the groups mentioned here welcome the competition, because they feel that it improves their practice and provides a stimulus to excellence.

CASE STUDY: EXAMPLE 2

A tabulation method can be used to analyze a departmental clientele network. The development of such a reference tool for the internal environment of the organization provides the manager with much information concerning relationships to be developed, aspects of the workflow to be considered, and regulations and guidelines that must be satisfied. The following is the clientele network of a spinal cord treatment service in a physical therapy department:

I. Clients
   A. Immediate clients
      1. Patients on the spinal cord injury service
      2. Hospital personnel assigned to the spinal cord injury service
   B. Secondary clients
      1. Family members
      2. Hospital medical staff for in-service education and clarification of policies and procedures
      3. Physical therapy students on clinical affiliation
      4. Local hospitals requesting information on special programs dealing with treatment of the spinal cord-injured patient
   C. Remote clients
      1. Local hospitals
      2. Home health agencies
II. Suppliers
   A. Resources
      1. Physicians within the hospital who refer patients to the spinal cord injury unit
      2. Medical supply companies that supply equipment for both the patients and the department
      3. Bureau of Vocational Rehabilitation to cover the cost of treatment and equipment
      4. Hospital transport system
   B. Associates
      1. National spinal cord treatment centers
      2. Other direct patient services, e.g., nursing, occupational therapy, speech, psychology, social service
      3. Home health agencies
      4. Professional journals
   C. Supporters
      1. Hospital physicians and residents
      2. Community service organizations
      3. Auxiliary organizations serving the spinal service
      4. Medical supply companies
      5. County Wheelchair Sports Association
      6. Public relations department of the hospital
III. Advisers
   A. Hospital administrators
   B. Other direct patient care services within the hospital

      C. Insurance companies
IV. Controllers
      A. Accreditation agencies
          1. Joint Commission on Accreditation of Hospitals (JCAH)
          2. Commission on Accreditation of Rehabilitation Facilities (CARF)
          3. Accrediting Council for Graduate Medical Education for Residency Program (CGME)
      B. Federal government
          1. Medicare reimbursement regulations
          2. Equal employment opportunity
          3. Working conditions
      C. State government
          1. Licensing regulations for physical therapists
          2. Medicaid reimbursement regulations
      D. County Hospital Association
      E. Professional associations' code of ethics
      F. Unions
      G. Hospital policies
V. Adversaries
      A. Opponents and enemies
          1. Consumer groups
          2. Hospital personnel resistant to change
      B. Rivals and competitors
          1. Other local rehabilitation centers sharing the same clientele network

---

NOTES

1. Bertram Gross, *Organizations and Their Managing* (New York: The Free Press, a Division of Macmillan Publishing Co. 1968), p. 114.

2. Ibid.

3. Ibid., p. 119–121.

4. Ibid. p. 121.

5. Ibid., p. 122.

6. Ibid., p. 130.

Chapter 16

Organizational Survival Strategies

CHAPTER OBJECTIVES

1. Identify the need for organizational survival as a fundamental goal of organizational effort.
2. Identify selected management strategies that are used to foster organizational survival: bureaucratic imperialism; cooptation; hibernation and adaptation; goal succession, expansion, and multiplication.
3. Identify the phases in the organizational life cycle that reflect major changes.
4. Relate the phases of the organizational life cycle to the functions of the manager.
5. Identify the organizational change process.
6. Relate the actions of the manager as change agent to the change process.
7. Identify specific strategies for initiating change in organizations.

Organizational survival and growth are implicit organizational goals, requiring the investment of energy and resources. Normally, only higher levels of management need give attention to organizational survival; it may be taken for granted by most members of the institution, who may even take action that threatens survival (e.g., a prolonged strike). There may be an unwillingness to admit the legitimacy of the survival goal because of its seeming self-serving aspect. Managers disregard the concept of organizational (including departmental and unit) survival only at their peril, however.

So fundamental is the goal of organizational survival that it underpins all other goals. Fostering this goal contributes to the satisfaction of the more explicit goals of the group or organization. Bertram Gross described this implicit goal as "the iron law of survival." The unwritten law of every organization, he said, is that its survival is an absolute prerequisite for its serving any interest whatsoever.[1]

Survival is articulated as a goal in certain phases of organizational development. The clientele network includes the specific categories of competitors, rivals, enemies, and opponents that must be faced. Certain threats to organizational survival may be identified:

- lack of strong, formal leadership after the early charismatic leadership of the founders
- too rapid change either within or outside the organization
- shifting client demand, with either the loss of clients or with the exercise of control by clients
- competition from stronger organizations
- high turnover rate in the rank and file or the leadership
- failure to recognize and accept organizational survival as a legitimate, although not the sole, organizational purpose

These factors drain from the organization the energy that should be goal-directed.

An organization ensures its survival through certain strategies and processes, such as bureaucratic imperialism, cooptation, patterns of adaptation, goal multiplication and expansion, organizational roles, limiting conflict, and integration of the individual into the organization. Astute managers recognize such patterns of organizational behavior and assess them realistically. A weak organization or unit cannot pull together the money, resources, and power to serve clients effectively.

BUREAUCRATIC IMPERIALISM

Organizations develop to foster a particular goal, serve a specific client group, or promote the good of a certain group. In effect, an organization stakes out its territory. Thus, a professional association seeks to represent the interests of members who have something in common, such as specific academic training and professional practice. A hospital or home health agency seeks to serve a particular area. A union focuses on the needs of one or several categories of worker. A political party attempts to bring in members who hold a particular political philosophy. A government agency seeks to serve a specific constituency.

The classic definition of bureaucratic imperialism reflects the idea that a bureaucratic organization exerts a kind of pressure first to develop a particular client group and then to expand it. It becomes imperialistic in the underlying power struggle and competition that ensues when any other group seeks to deal with the same clients, members, or area of jurisdiction. Matthew Holden, Jr. coined the term *bureaucratic imperialism* and defined it in the context of federal government agencies that must consider such factors as clients to be served, political aspects to be assessed, and benefits to be shared among administrative officials and key political clients. According to Holden's definition of the concept, bureaucratic imperialism is "a matter of interagency conflict in which two or more agencies try to assert permanent control over the same jurisdiction, or in which one agency actually seeks to take over another agency as well as the jurisdiction of that agency."[2] The idea of agency can be expanded to include any organization, the various components of the clientele network can be substituted for the constituency, and the role of manager can replace that of the administrative politician in those organizations that are not in the formal political setting.

Managers in many organizations can recognize the elements of this competitive mode of interaction among organizations. There may even be such competition among departments and units within an organization. In the health care field, competition may be seen in the areas of professional licensure and practice, accrediting processes for the organizations as a whole, the delineation of clients to be served, and similar areas.

Professional licensure has the effect of annexing specific "territory" as the proper domain of a given professional group, but other groups may seek to carry out the same, or at least similar, activities. For example, there is the question of the role of chiropractic in traditional health care settings. Is the use of radiological techniques the exclusive jurisdiction of physicians and trained radiological technicians, or should the law be changed to permit chiropractors greater use of these techniques? Psychiatrists question the expanding role of others who have entered the field of mental health. As each health care profession develops, the question of jurisdiction emerges.

The accrediting process in health care reflects similar struggles for jurisdiction. Which shall be the definitive accreditation process for mental health facilities, that approved by the American Psychiatric Association or that approved by the Joint Commission on the Accreditation of Hospitals (JCAH)? Should all these processes be set aside, leaving state governments only to exercise such control through the licensure of institutions?

Other examples may be drawn from the health care setting. There is the jurisdictional dispute over blood banking between the American Red Cross and the American Association of Blood Banks, as well as the competition of health maintenance organizations (HMOs) with the more traditional Blue

Cross and Blue Shield plans and commercial medical insurance companies. The area of health care planning also reflects this territorial question; several agencies, including both government and private agencies, require hospitals and other health care institutions to submit to several sets of planning mandates.

Although the charitable nature of health care has been emphasized traditionally, the elements of competition and underlying conflict must be recognized. With shifts in patient populations and changes in each health care profession, health care managers must assess the effects of bureaucratic imperialism in a realistic manner. The competition engendered by bureaucratic imperialism and the resultant total or partial "colonization" of an organizational unit or client group may be functional. Holden noted that conflict not only forces organizational regrouping by clarifying client loyalty and wishes, but also sharpens support for the agency or unit that "wins." Furthermore, it disrupts the bureaucratic form from time to time, causing a healthy review of client need, organizational purpose, and structural patterns.

COOPTATION

Another method that organizations use to help ensure their survival is cooptation, an organizational phenomenon by which entities tend to adapt and respond to change. Philip Selznick described and labeled this process, which is viewed as both a cooperative and an adaptive process. He defined this cooperation plus adaptation as "an adaptive response on the part of the organization in response to the social forces in its environment; by this means, the organization averts threats to its stability by absorbing new elements into the leadership of the organization."[3] The organization, in effect, shares organizational power by absorbing these new elements. Selznick called it a realistic adjustment to the centers of institutional strength.[4]

Formal vs. Informal Cooptation

In formal cooptation, the symbols of authority and administrative burdens are shared, but no substantial power is transferred. The organization does not permit the coopted group to interfere with organizational unity of command. Normal bureaucratic processes tend to provide sufficient checks and balances on any coopted group, just as they tend to restrict the actions of managers. Through formal cooptation, however, the organization seeks to demonstrate its accessibility to its various publics.

In health care, the cooptation process is suggested by the practice of appointing "ordinary" citizens to the board of trustees. Community mental health centers and some neighborhood health centers tend to emphasize consumer/community representation; Health Systems Agencies (HSAs) include both providers and consumers in planning for health care on a regional or statewide basis. The formalization of nursing home ombudsmen or patient care councils are still another example of this process.

Professional associations in those disciplines that have technical-level practitioners have sought to open their governing processes in response to the growing strength of the technical-level group. Increases in numbers, greater degree of training, further specialization, and a general emphasis on the democratic process and provision of rights for all members have fostered changes in these associations. Without the cooperative adaptation to such internal changes, additional associations may have been formed, possibly weakening the parent organization.

When an organization seeks to deal less overtly with shifting centers of power and to maintain the legitimacy of its own power, cooptation may be informal in nature. For example, managers may meet unofficially with informally delegated representatives of clients, employees, or outside groups. Organizational leaders may deal regularly with some groups, but there are no visible changes in the official leadership structures. No new positions are created; committee membership remains intact. The emphasis is on the substance of power, not its symbolic forms, such as title, official appointment, or power to vote. Informal cooptation may be more important than formal cooptation because of its emphasis on true power, although each form serves its unique purpose. An organization can blend formal and informal cooptation processes, since they are not mutually exclusive.

Control of Coopted Groups

Although the coopted group could gain strength and attempt to consolidate power, this does not happen frequently for several reasons. First, the organization has the means of controlling participation. For example, only limited support may be given to the group; there may be no physical space, money, or staff available to give to the coopted group, or management could simply withhold support. Another possible course is to assign so much activity to the coopted group that it cannot succeed easily. Key leaders of the coopted group generally retain their regular work assignments, but now have in addition projects and tasks relating to their special causes. Coopted leaders also become the buffer individuals in the organization, since the group has placed its trust in them and looks for results faster than they can be produced. Such leaders may find their base of action eroded and their activity turning into a thankless task.

In a more Machiavellian approach, organizational authorities could schedule meetings at inconvenient hours or control their agenda in such a way that issues of significance to the coopted group are too far down on the list of discussion items to be dealt with under the time constraints. Absolute insistence on parliamentary procedure may also be used as a weapon of control; a novice in the use of Robert's *Rules of Order* is at a distinct disadvantage when compared with a seasoned expert.

The subtle psychological process that occurs in the coopted individual who is taken into the formal organization as a distinct outsider acts as another controlling measure. The person suddenly becomes, for this moment, one of the power holders and derives new status. Certain perquisites also are granted. Consumer representatives, for example, may find their way paid, quite legitimately, for special conferences or fact-finding trips to study a problem. The individual, in becoming privy to more data and sometimes to confidential data, may start to "see things" from the organization's point of view.

Certain subtle social barriers may make the coopted individual uncomfortable, even though they may not be raised intentionally and may be part of the normal course of action for the group. For example, a female, nonvoting representative of a constituency who has been invited to attend a portion of a board meeting at an exclusive downtown club where women are permitted only in special areas may well be overwhelmed when ushered into the suite where the power elite sit at a long table, portfolios closed, business seemingly concluded except for this final agenda item—her cause. Even an informal setting, such as a swimming party or golfing match, may be intimidating if the coopted person feels out of place.

Individuals representing pressure groups find that their own time and energies are limited, even if they desire power. Other activities continue to demand their energies. In addition, certain issues lose popularity, and pressure groups may find their power base has eroded. Finally, the agenda items that were causes of conflict may become the recurring business of the organization. The conflict may become routinized, and the structure to deal with it may become a part of the formal organization. In the collective bargaining process, for example, the union is a part of the organization, and its leaders have built-in protection from factors that erode effective participation. Labor union officials commonly have certain reductions in workload so that they may attend to union business, space may be provided for their offices or meetings, and they may seek meetings with management as often as executives seek sessions with them. Cooptation has occurred, but without a loss of identity of the coopted group. In health care organizations, consumer participation has become part of the organizations' continuing activity through the development of a more stable process for consumer input, such as the HSA and the community governing board models.

HIBERNATION AND ADAPTATION

To maintain its equilibrium, an organization must adapt to changing inputs. This adjustment may take a passive form of hibernation in which the institution enters a phase of retrenchment. Cutting losses may be the sensible option. If efforts to maintain an acceptable census in certain hospital units, such as obstetrics or pediatrics, are unsuccessful, there may be an administrative decision to close those units and concentrate on providing quality patient care in the remaining services. An organization may adjust or adapt to changing inputs more actively by anticipating them. Staff specialists may be brought in, equipment and physical facilities updated, and goals restated. Finally, the overall corporate form may be restructured as a permanent reorganization that formalizes the cumulative effects of changes. A hospital may move from private sponsorship to a state-related, affiliated status, or a health care center may become the base service unit for mental health/ mental retardation programs in the area.

The relationships among the concepts of hibernation, adaptation, and permanent change strategies can be seen in the following case history of a state mental hospital. After the state legislature cut the budget of all state mental hospitals, the institution director began to set priorities for services so that the institution could survive. The least productive departments were asked to decrease their staff. The rehabilitation department lost two aide positions. The institution director had to force the organization into a state of hibernation in order to accomplish some essential conservation of resources.

The director of rehabilitation services revised the department goals to improve the chances of departmental survival. After closing ancillary services, the director concentrated staff on visible areas of the hospital and asked them to make their work particularly praiseworthy. At the same time, the director emphasized the need to document services so that patients' progress in therapy programs could be demonstrated. The director adapted to the change in the organization.

The program changes proved successful. The director of the rehabilitation department consolidated the changes and modified the department's goals. Instead of offering periodic programs to adolescent, neurological, geriatric, and acute care patients, the staff would concentrate on acutely ill geriatric patients. The staff applied for funds that were available to treat this population. At the same time, the staff determined that the adolescent unit could benefit from their services. Although funds were shrinking, the staff serviced this unit because needs in that area were unmet. The director and the staff decided to apply for private funds to service neurological and acute care cases so that these programs could also continue. By adopting a combined strategy of hibernation and adaptation, with alternate plans for expansion, the department director was able to foster not only departmental survival, but, ultimately, departmental growth.

GOAL SUCCESSION, MULTIPLICATION, AND EXPANSION

Because an organization that effectively serves multiple client groups can attract money, materials, and personnel more readily than can one with a more limited constituency, leaders may seek actively to expand the original goals of the organization. In addition to the pressures in the organizational environment that may force the organization to modify its goals as an adaptive response, success in reaching organizational goals may enable managers to focus on expanded or even new goals. The terms *goal succession, goal expansion,* and *goal multiplication* are used to describe the process in which goals are modified, usually in a positive manner.

Amatai Etzioni described this tendency of organizations to find new goals when old ones have been realized or cannot be attained. In goal succession, one goal is reached and is succeeded by a new one.[5] Etzioni cited David Sill's analysis of the goal evolution of the Foundation for Infantile Paralysis (March of Dimes). Having achieved its goals of arousing public interest in infantile paralysis and raising money for research and assistance to its victims, the organization could have ceased operations. Instead, it continued to function through its network of volunteers, national leaders, and central staff to achieve a new goal: prevention of birth defects.[6]

Sometimes an organization takes on additional goals because the original goals are relatively unattainable. A church may add a variety of social services to attract members when the worship forms and doctrinal substance per se do not increase the church's membership. A missionary group may offer a variety of health care or educational services when its direct evangelical methods cannot be used. The original goal is not abandoned, but it is sought indirectly; more tangible goals of service and outreach succeed this primary goal.

Goal expansion is the process in which the original goal is retained and enlarged with variations. Colleges and universities expand their traditional educational goals to include continuing education. The JCAH continues to focus primarily on inpatient acute care hospital accreditation, but expands its standards and accreditation process to home care, outpatient, and emergency care units. A collective bargaining unit negotiates specific benefits for its workers and takes on the administrative processing of certain elements, such as the pension fund; the basic goal of improving the circumstances of the workers is retained and expanded beyond immediate economic benefits. Another example of goal expansion may be seen in the work of the Red

Cross. Organized to deal with disaster relief in World War I, it subsequently expanded its work to assist in coordinating relief from all disasters, regardless of cause. In all these examples, the basic goal is retained and the new ones derived from it; the new goals are closely related and are essentially extensions of the original goal.

Goal multiplication is also a process in which an original goal is retained and new ones added. In this case, however, the new goals reflect the organization's effort to diversify. Goal multiplication is often the natural outgrowth of success. A hospital may offer patient care as its traditional, primary goal. To this it may add the goal of education of physicians, nurses, and other health care professionals. Because excellence in education is frequently related to the adequacy of the institution's research programs, research subsequently may become a goal. The hospital may take on a goal of participating in social reform, seeking to undertake affirmative action hiring plans and to foster employment within its neighborhood. It may offer special training programs for those who are unemployed in its area or for those who are physically or mentally impaired. It may coordinate extensive social services in order to assist patients and their families with both immediate health care problems and the larger social and economic problems they face.

Similar examples can be found in the business sector. A large hotel-motel corporation, with its resources for dealing with temporary living quarters, may go into the nursing home industry or the drug and alcohol treatment facility business by offering food, laundry, and housekeeping services; it may even operate a chain of convalescent or of alcohol and drug rehabilitation centers itself. Several real estate firms might consolidate their efforts in direct sale of homes and then offer mortgage services as an additional program. Organizations take on a variety of goals as a means of diversification; resources are directed toward satisfaction of all the goals. Such multiplication of goals is seen as a positive state of organizational growth.

ORGANIZATIONAL LIFE CYCLE

Organizational change can be monitored through the analysis of an organization's life cycle. This concept is drawn from the pattern seen in living organisms. In management and administrative literature, the development of this model stems from the work of Marver Bernstein, who analyzed the stages of evolution and growth of federal independent regulatory commissions.[7] This model of the life cycle can be applied to advantage by any manager who wishes to analyze a particular management setting.

The organization is assessed, not in chronological years, but in phases of growth and development. No absolute number of years can be assigned to each phase, and any attempt to do so in order to predict characteristics would force and possibly distort the model. The value of organizational analysis by means of the life cycle lies in its emphasis on characteristics of the stages rather than the years. For example, the neighborhood health centers established in the 1960s under Office of Economic Opportunity sponsorship had a relatively short life span in comparison with the life span of some large urban hospitals that are approaching a century or more of service. Both types of organizations have experienced the phases of the life cycle, with the former having completed the entire phase through decline and—in its original form—extinction.

The phases of the organizational life cycle usually meld into one another, just as they do in the biological model. Human beings do not suddenly become adolescents, adults, or senior citizens; so, too, organizations normally move from one phase to another at an imperceptible rate with some blurring of boundaries. Finally, not every organization reflects in detail every characteristic of each phase. The emphasis is on the cluster of characteristics that are predominant at a specific time.

Gestation

In this early formative stage, there is a gradual recognition and articulation of need and/or shared purpose. This stage often predates the formal organization; indeed, a major characteristic of this period is the movement from informal to formal organization. The impetus for organizing is strong, since it is necessary to bring together in an organized way the prime movers of the fledgling organization, its members (workers), and its clients.

Leadership tends to be strong and committed, and members are willing to work hard. Members' identification with organizational goals is strong, because the members are in the unique situation of actualizing their internalized goals; in contrast, those who become part of the institution later must subsequently internalize the institution's objectives. Members of the management team find innovation the order of the day. Creative ideas meet with ready acceptance, since there is no precedent to act as a barrier to innovation. If there is a precedent in the parent organization, it may be cast off easily as part of the rejection of the old organization. A self-selection process also occurs, with individuals leaving if they do not agree with the form the organizational entity is taking. This is largely a flexible process, free of the formal resignation and separation procedures that come later.

Youth

The early enthusiasm of the gestational phase carries over into the development of a formal organization. Idealism and high hopes continue to dominate the psychological atmosphere. The creativity of the gestational period is channeled toward developing an organization that will be free of the problems of similar institutions. There is a strong camaraderie among the original group of leaders and members. Organizational patterns have a certain inevitability, however. If a creative new organization is successful, it is likely to experience an increase in clients that will force it to formalize policy and procedure rapidly in order to handle the greater demand for service.

Some crisis may occur that precipitates expansion earlier than planned. A health center may have a plan for gradual neighborhood outreach, for example, but a sudden epidemic of flu may bring an influx of clients before it is staffed adequately. Management must make rapid adjustments in clinic hours and staffing patterns to meet the demand for specific services and, at the same time, to continue its plan for comprehensive health screening. A center for the mentally retarded may schedule one opening date, but a court order to vacate a large, decaying facility may require the new center to accept the immediate transfer of many patients. Routine, recurring situations are met by increasingly complex procedures and rules. Additional staff is needed, recruited, and brought into the organization, perhaps even in a crash program rather than through the gradual integration of new members.

At this point, a new generation of worker enters the organization. These workers are one phase removed from the era of idealism and deeply shared commitment to the organization's goals. The organizational structure, e.g., workflow, job descriptions, line and staff relationships, and role and authority, is tested. For the newcomer brought in at the management level, formal position or hierarchical office is the primary base of authority. Other members of the management team, as the pioneers, know each other's strengths and weaknesses intimately, but these managers may need to test the newcomer's personal attributes and technical competence. Sometimes, because the new organization attempts to deal with some problem in an innovative manner, an individual health care practitioner is hired in a nontraditional role; not only the professional and technical competence of that individual, but also the managerial competence of that individual is tested.

Communication networks are essential in any organization. During an organization's youth, it is necessary to rely on formal communication, because the informal patterns are not yet well developed, except within the core group. This lack of an easy, anonymous, informal communication network forces individuals to communicate mainly along formal lines of authority. The core group may become more and more closed, more and more "in," relying on well-developed, secure relationships that stem from a shared history in the developing organization, while the newcomers form a distinct "out" group.

The jockeying for power and position may be intense. If managers hold an innovative office, those who oppose such creative organizational patterns may exert significant pressure to acquire jurisdiction or to force a return to traditional ways. Since there may be much innovation in the overall organizational pattern, managers have little or no precedent against which they can measure their actions.

Certain problems center on the implementation of the original plans. The planners may start to experience frustration with managers who enter the organization during this period of formalization. Perhaps the original plans need modification; perhaps the innovative, ideal approach of the original group is not working, largely because of the change in the size of the organization. The line managers find themselves in the difficult situation of seeming to fail at the task on the one hand and being unable to make the original planners change their view on the other. The promise of innovation becomes empty, however, if the original planners guard innovation as their prerogative and refuse to accept other ideas.

In the youth phase of an organization, more time must be devoted to orientation and similar formal processes of integrating new individuals into the organization. Certain difficulties may be encountered in recruiting additional supervisors and professional practitioners; for example, there may be no secure retirement funds, no group medical and life insurance, and no similar benefits that are predicated on long-term investments and large membership. Salary ranges may be modest in comparison with those of more established organizations simply because insufficient time has passed for the development of adequate resources. The strong normative sense of idealism may have a negative effect on potential workers, as well as a positive one; a certain dedication to the organization's cause may be an inherent expectation with a concomitant understanding, often implicit, that personnel work in the new organization without an emphasis on monetary reward.

Bernstein stressed the increased concern for organizational survival in this youthful stage. The organization may become less innovative, because it is not sure of its strength. It may choose to fight only those battles in which victory is certain. In the case of regulatory bodies, which were Bernstein's major focus, the businesses subject to regulation may be perceived as stronger than the agency itself. In a health care organization, the new unit may be treated as a stepchild of related health care institutions. A new community mental health center or a home care organization, for example, may have to choose between competing with older, traditional units within the parent organization and being completely independent, still competing for resources but with less legitimacy of claim. A struggle not unlike the classic parent-adolescent conflict may emerge. Thus, organizational energy may go into an internal struggle for survival rather than into serving clients and expanding goals.

If the client groups are well defined and no other group or institution is offering the same service, a youthful organization may flourish. A burn unit in a hospital may have an excellent chance of survival as an organization because of the specificity of its clients as compared, for example, with the chance of a general medical clinic's survival. A similar positive climate may foster the development of units for treatment of spinal cord injury or for rehabilitation of the hand as specialized services. In effect, a highly specialized client group may afford a unit or an organization a virtual monopoly with its attendant position of strength.

Middle Age

The multiple constraints on the organization at middle age are compounded by several factors. In addition to the external influences that shape the work of the organization, there are internal factors that must be dealt with, such as the organizational pattern, the growing bureaucratic form, the weight of decision by precedent, and an increasing number of traditions.

On the other hand, the organization also reaps many benefits from middle age. Many activities are routine and predictable; roles are clear; and communication, both formal and informal, is relatively reliable. These years are potentially stable and productive. There is a reasonable receptivity to new ideas, but middle age is not usually a time of massive or rapid change and disruption, even the positive disruption resulting from major innovation. The manager in an organization in its middle age performs the basic traditional management processes in a relatively predictable manner.

Periods of rejuvenation are precipitated by a variety of events. A new leader may act as a catalytic agent, bringing new vision to the organization; for example, the president of a corporation may push for goal expansion by introducing a new line of products, or an aggressive hospital administrator may push for the development of an alternate health care service model. Mergers and affiliations with new and developing health care institutional forms, such as the HMO, community mental health center, or home care program, may be the catalytic agent or event. Although primarily negative events, the fiscal chaos associated with bankruptcy or the loss of accreditation as a hospital may cause the organization to reassess its goals and restructure its form, thus giving itself a new lease on life.

Some external crisis or change of articulated values in the larger society may make the organization vital to that society once again. The emergence of alternate modes of communal living reflects individuals' search for a mode of living that combats the alienation of urban society; these organizations are revitalized because of this renewed need for shared living arrangements. The effect of war on the vitality of the military is an obvious example of crisis as a catalytic agent that causes a spurt of new growth for an organization. The growth of consumer and environmental agencies is another organizational response to change and/or crisis in the larger society.

In health care, family practice is developing as a specialty in response to patients' wishes for a more comprehensive, more personal type of medical care. The hospice concept for the terminally ill is gradually becoming an alternative to the highly specialized setting of the acute care hospital.

An organization may experience a significant surge of vitality because of some internal activity, such as unionization of workers. During the covert as well as the overt stage of unionization, management may take steps to "get the house in order," including greater emphasis on worker-management cooperation in reaching the fundamental goals of the organization. Service of strong client groups may become more active, both to focus attention on the institution's primary purpose and to mobilize client good will in the face of the potential adversary, i.e., the union. Such internal regrouping activities foster rejuvenation in the organization as an offshoot of their primary purpose, avoiding unionization or reducing its impact.

Legislation of massive scope, particularly at the federal level, may have a rejuvenating effect. The infusion of money into the health care system via Medicare and Medicaid is partly responsible for the growth of the long-term care industry, although population trends and sociological patterns for care of the aged outside of the family setting are contributing factors. The passage of the National Health Care Planning and Resource Development Act rejuvenated some of the existing health planning agencies; its gradual phasing out, of course, has had the opposite effect in some instances by forcing a decline in certain planning groups. Changes in state professional licensure laws, as in the case of the nurse-practitioner, the physician's assistant, or the physical therapist, may bring such professional groups into a season of new vigor.

The bureaucratic hierarchy protects managers who derive authority from a position that traditionally is well defined by the organization's middle age. Planning and decision making are shared responsibilities, subject to several hierarchical levels of review. The same events that may spur rejuvenation also may hurl the organization into a state of decline, the major characteristic of the final stage: old age.

Old Age/Decline

Staid routines, resistance to change, a long history of "how we do things," little or no innovation, and concern with survival are the obvious characteristics of an organization in decline. There may be feeble attempts to maintain the status quo or to serve clients in a minimal fashion, but the greater organizational energy is directed toward efforts to survive. If the end is inevitable, resources are guarded so that the institution can fulfill its obligations to its contractual suppliers and to its past and present employees (e.g., through vested pension funds, severance pay, and related termination benefits). There may even be a well-organized, overt process of seeking job placement for certain members of the hierarchy; time and resources may be made available to such individuals. Sometimes key individuals from the dying organization attempt to develop a new organization.

Because of its dwindling resources, the organization no longer may serve clients well, and all but the most loyal clients will look for other organizations. The organization in decline cannot attract new clients; the cycle is broken. Without clients, the organization cannot mobilize financial and political resources to maintain its physical facilities, expand services, respond to technological change, or remain in compliance with new licensure or regulatory mandates. The end may come swiftly with a decision to close and a specific plan to do so in an orderly way. For example, a department store might announce a liquidation sale that ends with the closing date. Only the internal details of closing need attention. As far as clients are concerned, the organization has died.

A final closing date may be imposed on an organization; in a bankruptcy, for example, the date may be determined in the course of legal proceedings. Legislation that initially establishes certain programs may include a termination date, although the date is more commonly set when legislation to continue funding the program fails. The changes in medical care evaluation under the Professional Standards Review Organizations (PSROs) and the Office of Economic Opportunity neighborhood health centers are examples in the health care field of programs that move into a state of decline or closure when funding is no longer available through federal legislation.

The closing decision may be a more passive one; there may be a gradual diminution of services and selective plant shutdowns and layoffs, as may occur in manufacturing corporations that rely primarily on military or space contracts. Bankruptcy is costly in economic and political terms in some cases, so the decision is implemented slowly. Indeed, it sometimes seems that no one actually made a decision in some institutions that decline. Because of its unpopularity, the decision to close certain services, such as health care services, may be made in a somewhat passive way; however, the seemingly gradual slipping away of clients and the deterioration or outright closing of urban hospitals may be accompanied by the emergence of competitive forms of health care, such as home care units, neighborhood health centers, mobile clinics, and community mental health centers.

Although some organizations actually cease to exist, others may pass to another form or come under new sponsorship. For example, some of the neighborhood health centers under Office of Economic Opportunity sponsorship were absorbed into other federal government systems of health clinics. Several major railroad divisions were reorganized under Amtrak or Conrail. Some hospitals that had been owned and controlled by religious orders became general community-based, nonprofit institutions. Some organizations seem only to change title and official sponsorship. The various forms of agencies for health care planning over a decade or so have included Regional Medical Programs, Regional Comprehensive Health Planning programs, the HSAs and the statewide health planning agencies; the organizational structure, not the total mandate, of these agencies has changed.

The managers in the declining organization may find themselves in a caretaker role that involves such difficult activities as allaying the anxiety of workers, monitoring contradictory formal and informal information about closing, and developing a plan for closing while continuing to give a modicum of service to the remaining clients. Managers must continue to motivate the workers without a traditional reward system, even in its most limited form. Staff may be reduced, and workers may seek to use up all benefits that they may lose if the organization closes (e.g., sick days, vacation days, and similar personal days). Line managers may be forced to absorb the hostility of the workers facing job loss. Finally, a personal decision must be made: stay to the end, or leave and cut theoretical losses.

Paradoxically, this may be a time of great opportunity for managers. Middle managers may have an opportunity to participate in activities outside their normal scope as the executive team grows thin. This may be the ideal time for middle managers to try their hands at related jobs, because failure may be ascribed to the situation rather than to their inexperience or even incompetence. Valuable experience may be gained, because this may also be a time of great creativity as the gestational phase begins for a new organization with its unique opportunities, challenges, and frustrations. The organizational phoenix rises—sometimes.

We now move from general survival of the total organization to the specifics of individual change strategies.

ORGANIZATIONAL CHANGE

Recognition of and response to organizational change is yet another survival strategy. The astute manager anticipates change and is, sometimes, an active change agent.

The Change Process

Organizational change is a process by which a person or group of persons develops a strategy for effecting change in a social system. The changes are deliberate and, if successful, fulfill predetermined long- and short-term goals. The organizational change is carried out by an individual change agent who spearheads the change process. The change agent may work alone initially, but eventually will require the support of a small group. Efforts to change a group with more power and prestige than the change agent group require the support of a higher echelon group or sponsor to make the change successful.

There is no single correct method to initiate organizational change; however, observation, description, reflection, and focus are all necessary components of the strategy-building process.[8] The change agent must monitor results and be aware of any new events or participants in the change process. Organizational change requires both observation and analytical skills, as well as a working knowledge of formal and informal power roles.

The change process is spiral. It begins on a small scale and assumes bigger proportions as more events can be linked to the desired goals (Figure 16–1). It includes the following steps:

1. assessment: evaluation of the formal and informal power systems, examination of individual and unit roles, and isolation of a problem.
2. focus: determination of the boundaries of the problem. At the same time, long- and short-term goals must be established. It is important to identify possible allies and resources that might promote the change process. Obstacles must also be studied.
3. strategy building: development of an approach by the change agent. The change agent or the support group initiates events that promote goal attainment. Strategies are analogous to a plan for action.
4. working through: repetition of the first three steps as many times as deemed necessary.
5. resolution: the end of the change process, a time to evaluate the effect of the changes.

Figure 16–1 Organizational Change Process

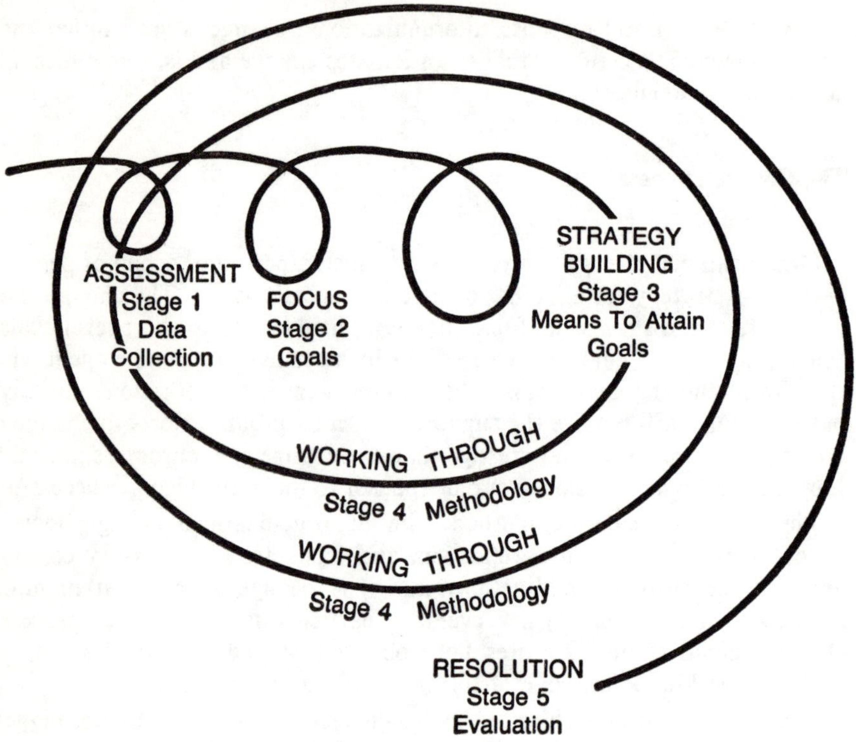

Because of its circular nature, the change process requires direction; therefore, success also depends on the methods selected to introduce the change
process. John Kotter and Leonard Schlesinger presented six strategies to
make change less threatening:[9]

1. *Education and communication*[10] are two easy ways to overcome resistance to change, since the logic of a change is understood before the
   process begins. Individual and group discussions, memos, and reports
   are used to open a communication network. This process is time-
   consuming and requires a good relationship between the initiators and
   the group affected by the change.
2. *Participation and involvement*[11] engages potential resistors in some aspect of the design and implementation of the change on the assumption

that involved participants become committed to the change. This strategy takes a great deal of time; furthermore, if not managed well, the strategy can produce poor results.

3. *Facilitation and support*[12] can foster new changes by dissipating fear and anger. This approach may be time-consuming and expensive. Even so, after energy has been expended in offering support, the change process may well fail.

4. *Negotiation and agreement*[13] can be used to offer incentives to active or potential resistors. The burden of adjustment is eased by trade-offs and negotiations. This strategy makes it possible to avoid major conflicts, but initiators might have to compromise.

5. *Manipulation of cooptation*[14] involves covert attempts to influence others by the selective use of information and the intentional structuring of events. Coopted individuals may become angry if they discover their endorsement is valued above their ideas. If handled poorly, manipulation can also foster distrust and increase resistance to change.

6. *Explicit and implicit concern*[15] can force change on subordinates if the change agent has sufficient power. This method is quick, but dissatisfied individuals may work to undermine the changes.

Change is resisted for four reasons: (1) lack of trust, (2) a different assessment of a situation, (3) a desire to protect the status quo, and (4) protection of self-interest.[16] Successful change strategies depend on careful assessment of the people who will be affected by the changes. The extent of the resistance should be determined by observation and the change process initiated again. The best strategy can then be selected.

Change is a part of life, but unregulated change in organizations can prove taxing and difficult for group relations. Organizational change is a planned process in which the social structure of the group is altered by formal or informal interaction. Social change can improve patient services and increase the status of allied health care professionals.

CASE STUDY: SEDENTARY PATIENTS IN A GERIATRIC FACILITY

Background: Shore Acres is a 125-bed health care facility owned by a corporation and managed by a health care administrator who is responsible for all the hospital functions (Figure 16–2). The Director of Nursing, a nurse-practitioner, oversees all direct patient services. Routine functions are carried out by nursing aides. The speech therapist, physical therapist, dentist, and activity director all report to the Director of Nursing.

Figure 16–2 Organizational Chart

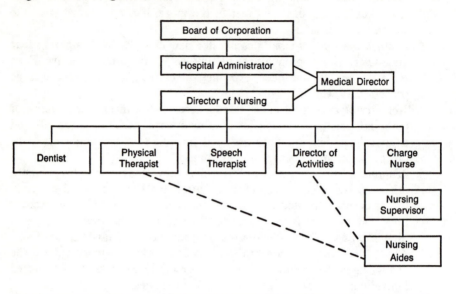

The Director of Nursing uses her power to control the other services. Because the Medical Director is a part-time employee, she is also influenced by the Director of Nursing.

Assessment

The speech therapist and physical therapist note that patients are frequently undressed and lying in bed. Both feel that this is detrimental to the patients' health, since elderly individuals lose functional skills if they do not keep moving.

Focus

The speech therapist and physical therapist would like to strengthen the rehabilitation program of the facility. They would like to introduce an occupational therapist into the hospital social system. Do you agree with the focus selected by the physical therapist and social worker? Can you generate another focus that would address the problem? The Director of Nursing would probably claim that she needed more staff to improve patient care. She might maintain that patients must remain in bed because she has so little help. Does this solution address the original problem?

Goals must be established for the change process, for example, "to keep patients engaged in activities." This goal would require the cooperation of the Director of Activities. Another goal might be "to increase functional independence of patients." This goal clearly identifies the self-care skills needed by patients. Select a goal and refine it. Break the goal into short-term pieces.

Strategy Building

What strategies would you use to accomplish the goal? Select a strategy from the six listed earlier and discuss whether each would work and why or why not. Who would need to help institute the change process? Which people might support the change, and which people might oppose the change?

The physical therapist decided to use the strategy of education and communication. The therapist met with the physician and discussed the problem. The physician was concerned and asked for the physical therapist's solution. The social worker used the same strategy to enlist the help of the Director of Activities. Once the physician and the Director of Activities were engaged in the change process, the group decided to include the Director of Nursing, using the participation and involvement strategy.

Working Through

The Director of Nursing used this opportunity to expand her staff. The change group encouraged her to hire two "rehabilitation aides." These two nursing aides would be supervised by the therapists. The Director of Nursing agreed to support the idea of hiring an occupational therapy consultant. This stage was advanced by the strategy of negotiation and agreement.

There are several more stages to working through the problem. The aides must be trained and the consultant hired. The group must again address the best strategy to keep the patients moving.

Resolution

This case study will be ended when the patient problem is solved. The group must use the new positions and resources to address the original problem.

Clearly, the change process can be initiated by an individual or a small group. The change may be planned by people who have no power, but the ultimate success of the change requires the support of a person or group who enjoys some power in the social system. Strategies are evaluated and adjusted during the working through stage, which is why feedback is so important. Change can improve social organizations if it is well conceived and executed.

NOTES

1. Bertram Gross, *Organizations and Their Managing* (New York: The Free Press, a Division of Macmillan Publishing Co., 1968), p. 454.

2. Matthew Holden, Jr., "Imperialism in Bureaucracy," *American Political Science Review* (December, 1966): 943.

3. Philip Selznick, *TVA and the Grass Roots* (New York: Harper Torchbooks, 1966), p. 13.

4. Ibid., pp. 13 and 260–261.

5. Amatai Etzioni, *Modern Organizations* (Englewood Cliffs, NJ: Prentice-Hall, 1964), pp. 13–14.

6. David L. Sills, *The Volunteers* (Glencoe, IL: The Free Press, 1957), p. 64, cited in Etzioni, *Modern Organizations*, p. 13.

7. Marver Bernstein, *Regulating Business by Independent Commission* (Princeton, NJ: Princeton University Press, 1955).

8. Virginia Schein, "Individual Power and Political Behaviors in Organizations: An Inadequately Explored Reality," *The Academy of Management Reviews* 2 (1977): 64–72.

9. John P. Kotter and Leonard A. Schlesinger, "Choosing Strategies for Change," *Harvard Business Review* (1979): 106–114.

10. Ibid., p. 109.

11. Ibid.

12. Ibid., p. 110.

13. Ibid.

14. Ibid.

15. Ibid.

16. Ibid., p. 111.

Chapter 17

Personal, Work Group, and Organizational Conflict

CHAPTER OBJECTIVES

1. Define conflict from three perspectives: personal, work group, and organizational.
2. Identify the significance of the study of conflict in the organizational setting.
3. Understand the origins of conflict situations.
4. Develop strategies for analyzing each type of conflict.
5. Learn to deal with personal, small group, and organizational conflict.
6. Analyze organizational conflict in terms of its causes, participants, and processes.
7. Identify strategies for dealing with conflict in organizations.

Conflict is an inevitable component of cooperative action. The effects of conflict are felt by all participants in organizational life; no one is immune to conflict, be it personal, small group/work group, or organizational. By its nature, organizational life consists of carefully orchestrated conflict, so much so that one of the classic functions of a manager is that of coordination, which includes promoting cooperation and minimizing conflict.

Dictionary definitions of conflict range from terms such as variance, incompatibility, disagreement, and inner divergence to controversy, opposing sides, and rivalry. Conflict may be defined as a struggle among clashing interests, values, or ideas that disturbs an existing equilibrium. It is a state of external and internal tension that results when two or more demands are made on an individual, group, or organization.

Examples of conflict follow:

• patient's need for further care versus limits on eligibility under particular payment status

- scheduling of aides and transporters when more than one unit (e.g., physical therapy, nuclear medicine, radiology) seeks priority in patient transport

- employee unwilling to accept schedule readjustments for evening and weekend coverage because of personal commitments outside the usual work hours

- directives issued by state government regulatory agency for health and counterpart agency for welfare on certain aspects of patient eligibility for care and on institutional licensure or program participation

- personal health care philosophy of individual practitioner versus that espoused by organization

SIGNIFICANCE OF THE STUDY OF CONFLICT

The health care practitioner might react negatively to the whole idea of conflict, musing "I did not come to this organization to fight; I came to give patient care; I am not in the business of conflict." The manager and health care practitioner must understand the phenomenon of conflict within organizations, however, so that they can make it acceptable, predictable, and, therefore, manageable. Conflict must be accepted as an inevitable part of all group effort. The causes of conflict are located primarily in the organizational structure with its system of authority, roles, and specialization. The clash of personal styles of interaction can be analyzed with the intent of dealing more effectively with such clashes. Conflict can be accepted as an element of change, a positive catalyst for continual challenge to the organization. Aggression may be accepted and channeled to foster survival.

If conflict is not channeled and controlled, it may have negative effects that impede the growth of both the individual and the organization. If conflict is unlimited, the institution may be destroyed; for example, a prolonged, unresolved strike may cause a company eventually to go out of business. If the organization is in a hibernation or an expansion phase in its life cycle with all its energies focused in one area, intense conflict or strong competition may be disastrous, because such an organization has limited, if any, resources to offset the negative effects of conflict. If both participants are strong, the conflict may result in mutual annihilation.

In certain situations, on the other hand, conflict has positive effects; it may clarify relationships, effect change, and define organizational territory or jurisdiction. When there has been an integrative solution, resulting from open review of all points of view, agreement is strengthened and morale heightened. Conflict tends to energize an organization, forcing it to keep alert, to plan and anticipate change, and to serve clients in more effective ways.

Conflict in some of its aspects has a certain dramaturgical value, as in the catharsis of a strike or riot. Militant behavior by a protest group or a union is a show of power, an indication of the group's strength, or a tangible demonstration of its activity on behalf of its members. Confrontation may be needed to effect some long overdue reform. Some health care professionals have found that a strike has been the only means of obtaining the necessary equipment or reasonable staffing patterns to provide proper patient care.

PERSONAL CONFLICT

Defined as "a particular form of frustration involving an internal stress which results from the simultaneous arousal of two incompatible response tendencies that are similar to the kinds of tendencies elicited by positive and negative reinforcers,"[1] personal conflicts are mental battles that are part of everyday life. The conflict arises from frustration and is resolved by learning a way to satisfy all conflicting desires. Rewards may be positive or negative, but the learning occurs in any case because the outcome reinforces future behavior.

Personal conflict is a polarity of antagonistic forces that can be examined from several perspectives:

- Sigmund Freud and Carl Jung regarded inner conflict as a part of the personality.
- Erik Erikson proposed eight developmental stages that must be resolved by every individual. If not, the result of each stage is carried over into the next level that must then be resolved.
- Neal Miller and John Dollard developed a reinforcement theory to explain conflict behavior by graphing responses to conflict.
- Kurt Lewin established a typology that presents conflict as positive and negative forces in a field.

The Polarity of Conflict

According to Freud, who viewed the mind as an open system, incoming energy creates an imbalance and upsets the individual's equilibrium. The resulting inner tensions generate psychic energy that produces conflict. The greater the inequities in energy, the greater the tension. The person experiences the anxiety of conflict. Once the opposing forces are resolved, equilibrium is restored.

Jung believed that conflicting tendencies formed the basis of life because polar elements both attract and repel each other. Some personality polarities are introversion versus extroversion, thinking versus feeling, and love versus hate. The stable personality recognizes the polar forces and works to integrate both sides.

Because people have polar forces, one-sided solutions to conflicts must be avoided. Unfortunately, it is common to label conflict as a battle—one force competing with another for the same resources. This military analogy reinforces the concept of the win/lose approach. This is a primitive way to resolve conflicts, because the loser will work to regain lost resources. Because the losing side is not represented in the resolution, the loser's needs will become important once again, and the conflict will require additional attention.

Conflict in Infancy

Babies are too helpless to manipulate objects and satisfy their own inner desires. Because they can express their needs only in a limited way, they are dependent on their care-givers. Frustration builds if an infant wants something and the desire is not understood by the care-giver. The baby may also be frustrated by a desire to act in a way that is inconsistent with the care-giver's goals.

Infants have a distorted view of the world. Their external and internal worlds are merged; mother, other people, and the environment are all one. Infants are narcissistic and consider everything an extension of themselves. Hungry babies cannot rationalize that hunger is a temporary condition; instead, they believe the entire world feels miserable and hungry. On the other hand, satiated infants regard the world in a positive way. The fusion of self, others, and the environment continues until infants can express their needs. Then, they slowly learn that their care-givers are not part of themselves.

Freud and Jung emphasized the importance of early learning. To Freud, the stable individual must balance or check the forces that operate in the personality; the exact nature of the balance is determined by early influences on the developing individual.[2] Jung regarded the personality as an energy system that could be altered by outside events. "Tension, conflict, stress and strain are all feelings that arise from imbalances in the psyche."[3] The greater the inequities among the structures, the greater the feeling of tension or conflict. The influence of early learning on a person's later interpretation of life events was emphasized by both Freud and Jung. Conflict is a normal feeling because no one has totally congruent desires. Early influences and the polar nature of conflict can be seen in the following example:

Jane was taught to be neat. Sloppy work habits were disparaged by her parents and teachers. Although Jane professes to be neat, her house is always cluttered and disorganized. Periodically, Jane attacks the mess and cleans thoroughly, which takes her about a week of work. Once order has been restored, Jane relaxes, and the clutter slowly reappears. When the mess becomes bothersome again, Jane's conflict about work habits reappears. Her inner tension builds until she cleans up the clutter. The cleaning restores her feelings of orderliness, and her inner conflict creates less tension. To break the cycle, Jane must examine her feelings about orderliness and the expectations of her parents and teachers.

Developmental Perspective

Erikson expanded Freud's theory of personality development, dividing a life span into eight stages. Each stage is a target for personal conflict. Individuals can work through each stage or carry unresolved issues into the next stage of life. Because the effective resolution of each stage requires a balance among polar forces, some conflicts are longstanding and reappear throughout a person's life. The stages are

1. trust vs. mistrust (0–1 year)
2. autonomy vs. shame (1–3 years)
3. initiative vs. guilt (4–5 years)
4. industry vs. inferiority (6–11 years)
5. identity vs. role diffusion (12–18 years)
6. intimacy vs. isolation (young adult)
7. generativity vs. stagnation (middle age)
8. ego identity vs. despair (aging)[4]

The following example helps to demonstrate the stages:

George is a 40-year-old man who has not resolved the initial conflict of trust versus mistrust. George distrusts everyone. He has no friends and regards people with suspicion. His interactions are guarded and defensive. This unresolved conflict is part of George's personality. All of the other stages have been affected by his failure to resolve the initial stage.

Conflicts can be traced to the failure to work through these stages at an age-appropriate time. Maturity requires work at every stage. Freud, Jung, and Erikson all agree that unresolved conflicts remain with the person, appearing again and again throughout life in a variety of forms.

Conflict and Learning

Other theorists study conflict from an external vantage point. Two of these theorists, Miller and Dollard, developed an explanation of conflict that is based on psychoanalytic theory, C.L. Hull's formulations on learning, and information from social anthropology. They theorized that personal conflict emerges from unconscious emotions that are incongruous with other feelings. The basis for these feelings may be traced to the parent's handling of four major situations: feeding, toileting or cleanliness training, early sex education, and training to control anger and aggression.[5] The social context for human behavior was also considered important.

Basically, Miller and Dollard viewed response to conflict as the formation of a habit, e.g., a link between stimulus and response,[6] and they emphasized the conditions that formulate or dissolve habits.[7] Pavlov's dogs learned to link the sound of a bell with food, salivating when they heard a bell even if food was not offered as a reward. This response to a bell became a habit.

Miller and Dollard represented conflict in terms of five assumptions based on their application of Hull's work on learning theory to human situations. Behavior was analyzed on a gradient where the left side is time or distance from the goal and the bottom is the strength of the stimulus. The assumptions developed by Miller and Dollard are

1. The tendency to approach a goal becomes stronger the nearer the individual is to the goal (the gradient of approach).
2. The tendency to avoid a negative stimulus becomes stronger the nearer the individual is to the stimulus (the gradient of avoidance).
3. The gradient of avoidance is steeper than the gradient of approach.
4. An increase in the drive associated with the approach or avoidance raises the general level of the gradient.
5. If there are two competing responses, the stronger will occur.[8]

Learning theorists identify four types of conflict:

1. approach-approach conflict when "the individual is confronted with two desirable but incompatible goals"[9]
2. approach-avoidance conflict when "a single object, person, or situation has both attracting and repelling attributes"[10]
3. a double approach-avoidance conflict in which there are alternative possibilities, each possessing positive and negative characteristics[11]

4. avoidance-avoidance conflicts when "the individual must choose between two undesirable courses of action"[12]

The analysis of behavior manifested by animals who experienced conflict as a
result of experimental manipulation offers insight into human behavior. To
solve an approach-approach conflict, animals usually select one of the
favorable alternatives. Approach-avoidance conflicts produce vacillating behavior. Double approach-avoidance conflicts produce immobility. Finally,
avoidance-avoidance conflicts create so much anxiety that animals block or
fail to respond.[13]

The uncertainty of the approach-avoidance conflict can be depicted on a
gradient. Miller and Dollard usually plotted the distance from the goals or
time against the goal. Conflict arises when the strength of the tendency to
approach is countered by the strength of the tendency to avoid the stimulus.
The subjects must use additional mental energy to break the deadlock, or
personal conflict.[14] The following is an example of how learning affects conflict behavior:

> Joe is punished every time he puts his elbows on the table during
> dinner. His father lifts Joe's arm and bangs Joe's elbow on the
> table if Joe does not remove his arm. Joe rarely forgets to keep his
> elbows off the table. Joe, however, is more comfortable with his
> elbows on the table. Joe experiences an approach-avoidance conflict
> every time he sits down at the dinner table. He responds to the
> anxiety by eating rapidly and does not linger at the table.
>
> Joe may displace the anger he feels toward his father onto anoth-
> er object or person. Joe may kick a chair if he is angry with his
> father. He knows the consequences of hitting his father; therefore,
> he chooses to kick a chair.

Diagramming Conflict

Lewin tried to classify behavior in the context of the environment by
examining the similarities, differences, and relationships among the parts of
a conflict situation. He defined conflict as a force that acts on a person and
diagrammed the psychological forces that create a conflict. These forces may
push in opposite directions and be equal in strength.[15]

Lewin lists three types of personal conflict. These can be compared to the
four areas of conflict presented by Miller and Dollard.

1. Approach-approach conflict
2. Approach-avoidance conflict
3. Double approach-avoidance conflict

4. Avoidance-avoidance conflict

Although Lewin's categories were used by Miller and Dollard, Lewin's approach to conflict is unique. (For a detailed description of his work and drawings, consult *A Dynamic Theory of a Personality,* 1935.) His ideas are simplified in the following series of diagrams:

1. approach-approach

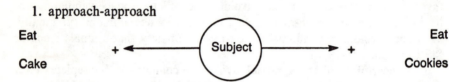

Subject can approach either choice. The person usually selects one of the two positive choices.

2. approach-avoidance

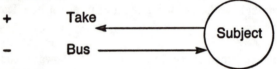

Subject is usually ambivalent because both choices have positive and negative outcomes. Some force tips the decision in one direction or the other.

3. double approach-avoidance

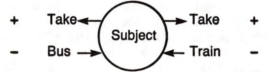

Subject is usually ambivalent because both choices have positive and negative factors. Some force tips the decision in one direction or the other.

4. avoidance-avoidance

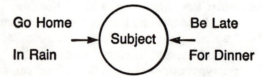

Subject avoids the decision because both outcomes are unsatisfactory.

Diagramming the personal conflict can increase an individual's understanding of a situation.

Resolution of Personal Conflict

There are a number of ways to resolve personal conflict. An individual can accept one alternative or the other, reject one alternative or the other, or try to combine positive and negative forces in a solution. Lewin developed a method to unify conflicting forces called a Force Field Analysis.[16]

The person who is experiencing conflict generates objective data to acquire an overview of the situation and resolve the conflict. The six stages of the process are

1. Schedule a period of uninterrupted time to study the personal conflict.
2. List all the forces pushing in one direction. Repeat the process for all the forces pushing in the opposite direction.
3. Read over the list and label the forces as positive or negative.
4. Take another sheet of paper and divide the paper in half. Put the positive forces on one side and the negative forces on the other side. Look over the list and refine the labeling system by dividing the positive forces into very positive forces (++), positive forces (+), and barely positive forces (−+). Divide the negative forces into very negative (−−), negative (−), or barely negative (+−).
5. Recopy the list and group the forces into similar categories, e.g., all the (++) forces in the same area, all the (+−) forces in another.
6. Put the list away for a period of time, even if only for an hour or so. Bring the list out and weigh the positive and negative forces. Determine which categories balance and which categories create the difference needed to make a decision.

The following example might help explain the process:

Gloria struggled with a decision. Should she continue her education and attend graduate school? She vacillated for several weeks and decided to try to analyze her options. She set aside an hour to study her personal conflict (Step 1). She listed all of the forces that pushed her in one direction or the other (Step 2). Gloria then divided the forces into positive and negative categories (Step 3). She further divided the forces into three degrees of positive or negative strength (Step 4, Exhibit 17-1). She recopied this list and grouped the similar categories (Step 5, Exhibit 17-2). Gloria put the list away for several days and then brought the list out again (Step 6).

Exhibit 17-1 Goal: Decision Regarding Graduate School (Step 4)

Positive		Negative	
Pursue knowledge	(+)	Pressure of school	(−)
Better credentials	(++)	Expense of education and fees	(−−)
Impress Mom and Dad	(+−)	No salary coming in for one year	(−−)
Earn more money	(++)	Possible loss of friendships	(−+)
Meet new people	(+)	Parents cannot offer money to help	(−+)
Time to reflect on future	(+−)	Cannot own a car	(−−)
Avoid responsibility for working full time	(+−)		
Campus life	(+)		

Exhibit 17-2 Goal: Decision Regarding Graduate School (Step 5)

Positive		Negative	
Earn more money	(++)	Expense of education and fees	(−−)
Better credentials	(++)	No salary coming in for one year	(−−)
		Cannot own a car	(−−)
Pursue knowledge	(+)		
Meet new people	(+)	Pressure of School	(−)
Campus life	(+)		
Impress Mom and Dad	(+−)	Possible loss of friendships	(−+)
Avoid responsibility for working full time	(+−)	Parents cannot offer money to help	(−+)
Time to reflect on future	(+−)		

Gloria analyzed her conflict and realized that she wanted to go to graduate school but did not want to lose any more time or money. She decided to compromise, and she enrolled in a part-time evening graduate program. This compromise solution included all of the forces that Gloria listed.

SMALL GROUP CONFLICT

A small group consists of two or more individuals who share some goal or purpose. The shared goal generates interdependence. A group is not an aggregate of people but individuals who communicate and modify their behavior in light of the behavior of others.[17] For example, a collection of individuals who are riding in an elevator is an aggregate of people; the riders have no commitment or interaction. If, however, the elevator stops between floors, the individuals will form a group; they become interdependent and share a goal.

Every small group is unique and has a collective personality that depends on all the individuals in the group. Thus, if one member is happy, sad, or absent, the composition of the collective personality changes. The collective group experience is called the group culture.[18]

Groups are part of daily life. Children participate in family and play groups. Adults move into a variety of groups, since they are members of a work, recreation and self-care groups. Thus, groups are common at home, leisure, and work.

Small groups may contain as few as 2 or as many as 20 members.[19,20] Although group members may see themselves as positive, cooperative, and friendly, they frequently act in negative, uncooperative, and unfriendly ways. Group life is not always pleasant. At times, group members experience emotions that create anxiety, and these emotions can build up and create group conflict. Group conflict is commonplace and endemic to group life.

Origin

Conflict began with Adam and Eve as they struggled with the forbidden fruit. Since ancient times, humans have known the limitations of a solitary existence. Our ancestors relied on each other for food, protection, nurturance, and kinship. Survival depended on group membership; banishment proved a severe punishment. Today, opportunities for a solitary existence are limited. In fact, because of increased population, sophisticated means of travel and communication, and advances in technology, modern lives are interdependent. Few individuals are capable of independent living. Instead, people are trained to perform in only one or two specialized areas; they purchase other services. Thus, daily living requires individuals to interface with a number of other individuals and groups. Because group life is not always harmonious, individuals must learn to cope with group conflict.

Many negative comments are made about group life because "man seems to be a herd animal who is often in trouble with his herd."[21] The push to satisfy the personal desires of the group members must be tempered by the pull to fulfill societal obligations. The I struggles with the demands of we. The I does not, however, wish to be outcast. Thus, people struggle with dual desires—to satisfy personal desires and to satisfy group demands. Conflict arises when personal needs are overrun by the group needs.

Feelings also color an individual's view of reality. People see, hear, smell, taste, and feel differently. Thus, an enjoyable incident for John creates stress and anxiety for Kathy. Group conflict on this basis, which is not uncommon, originated in childhood experiences.

Types of Group Conflict

There are three types of group conflict. Conflicts may be based on resource allocation, ideological differences, or perceived threats to personal identities.[22] At times, the cause of a particular conflict cannot be clearly identified. The issues are merged, and the conflict is complex. Resource-based conflicts are difficult to resolve, but some progress toward resolution is possible. Resolution of cognitive conflicts may be more elusive because ideas cannot be destroyed; thoughts may hibernate and later reappear.

Theoretical Perspectives

Group conflict can be explained from several theoretical perspectives: (1) psychoanalytical, (2) developmental, and (3) systems approaches. Each perspective offers a unique focus for the study of conflict.

Psychoanalytical Approach

Those who adhere to the psychoanalytical approach believe that the group struggles between task and emotional needs. This can be pictured as a wheel divided into two halves. If the group energy shifts, the wheel is unbalanced; the group moves to establish a new balance. The shifts are based on both conscious and unconscious desires that emerge from infancy. Tension arises from unmet needs on either level. The most productive goals satisfy the emotional and task needs of members. A goal that deals only with task or only with emotions cannot fulfill the members' needs. Psychoanalytical theory can be used to explain some complex aspects of small group life, such as dependency, intimacy, boundaries, authority, conscious and unconscious feelings.

W.C. Schutz[23] presented three areas of interpersonal need that are addressed by groups: inclusion, control, and affection. Groups develop in stages as members work together on group goals. The group deals initially with membership issues (inclusion), authority issues (control), and attraction among members (affection) in that order. These three issues are reversed in importance as the group matures.

Wilfred R. Bion[24] also addressed the unconscious motives of group members. He noted that the group's basic emotional issues, i.e., fight-flight, pairing, and dependency, are counterbalanced by ego-directed work. In fight-flight, group members fight to keep their identity separate from that of the group. This feeling then changes to flight as members flee from the task. Excessive eating, peripheral discussions, and small talk are examples of flight behavior. The task is at times so stressful that members fight to keep their egos separated from the group. Flight, or a refusal to address the task, offers another refuge from the emotionality of the group.

In pairing, group members watch as one or two pairs interact; the unconscious motive is a deep-seated desire for a leader to emerge from the paired interaction. Dependent behavior is frequently viewed, as members complain about the dearth of leadership, the shortcomings of the task, or the leaders' lack of abilities. These conscious or unconscious motives must be checked by the members' commitment to work. Work requires a balance of member needs so that the task and emotional issues are addressed equally.

Developmental Approach

Developmental group theorists conclude that groups go through stages of development. Tuchman presented the following model:[25]

1. Groups initially concern themselves with orientation, which is accomplished by testing. This is the exploration of dependency relationships and preexisting standards.[26]
2. The second stage is characterized by conflict and polarization around interpersonal issues. The individual members resist the group's influence and task requirements.
3. In the third stage, the members develop a cohesive feeling, and new standards and roles are adopted. To promote task, or the goal of the group, intimate opinions are expressed. Harmony is important.
4. Finally, the group is able to use their roles to achieve the goals of the group. Roles become flexible, and group energy is devoted to the task.

Developmental theorists cite the importance of conflict and regard the struggle as a stage of growth. The group can evolve if members address their individual differences.

Systems Approach

Lewin developed a *systems approach* to explain group behavior by addressing the forces that shape individual and group behavior. Lewin stressed the importance of subjective interpretations of live events. Actions cannot be viewed as isolated events, because the individual is part of a social system.

People exist in a life space that is a psychological environment; it represents the world as the person experiences it. Individual behavior is determined by all the possible facets that comprise the life space. The life space is divided into regions that are differentiated from the background, *valences* (degree of attraction to a goal) that promote or retard movement, *barriers* that impede movement in the life space, and *forces* that are either internal or external pressures to move. Conflict can be viewed as forces or barriers that impede or promote movement toward a valence or goal.

The system seeks balance or equilibrium. Lewin's focus on the entire social system and his view of the importance of understanding everyone's subjective experience are useful concepts. Change can be viewed as an event that upsets the equilibrium of the system. The group is an open system, receiving input from the environment. The group needs feedback or information that is fed into the system to keep the system on course.

Resolution of Small Group Conflict

The first step in resolving group conflict is to identify the underlying causes and categorize the conflict as a resource, ideological, or personal identity conflict. If there are multiple causes, the components of the conflict that can be linked to each category should be identified.

People react to conflict in a variety of ways. Some reactions are unconscious and difficult to address. Other reactions are conscious and promote conflict resolution.

Unconscious Resolution Methods

There are several unconscious means to protect the ego from anxiety-producing events. These strategies are called defense mechanisms:

- Repression is a method of pushing unpleasant thoughts or feelings into the unconscious. The person may feel a vague pull when reminded of them, but the cause is hidden from the conscious. For example, Fred claims that he loves to play golf and plays with his boss every week. After Fred changed jobs, he never touched his golf clubs.

- Rationalization is a substitution process by which acceptable thoughts or feelings are substituted for unacceptable ones. For example, Alice claims she loves to attend staffing meetings, although she always comes late and leaves early.

- Denial is a refusal to admit that a conflict or problem exists. It is a form of repression, because the unpleasant thoughts and emotions are negated. For example, Matilde is always shouting at John during meetings. When asked about her behavior, however, Matilde claims that she never shouts at anyone.

- Projection is a method of moving the cause of anxiety from the inner world to a person or event in the external world. For example, Howard refuses to come to the executive council meeting, claiming that no one will listen to him.

These defense mechanisms create communication barriers, because they make it difficult to share deep-seated emotions and thoughts. Unconscious thoughts obviously cannot be tapped as easily as conscious thoughts and emotions. There are a variety of training courses that can be used to teach people how to move unconscious blocks into conscious integrating experiences, however.

If a group conflict continues without any sign of abatement, the issues may be unconscious. Resolution may require the intervention of a trained facilitator, or the group leader must be given the responsibility of conflict resolution.

Conscious Resolution Methods

There are two conscious strategies to promote conflict resolution: compromise and integration. Compromise requires interaction and an agreement to work together. It is a mutual agreement to solve the differences by concessions on both sides. Since each side gives up something, there is no loser. Individuals who are familiar with competition may consider compromise a surrender, which opens them to dangerous concessions. This view is a short-sighted and pessimistic view of compromise.

Compromise can be a creative solution to the cause of the conflict. Group members share ideas and together they alter their concerns. This sharing is the strength of group interaction.

Integration is the most difficult method of resolving conflicts. Instead of making concessions in a compromise, individuals unite their differences in the solution. Successful integration requires group members who express their task and emotional needs, are able to set priorities in their issues and concerns, are willing to work on a method to integrate polar desires and needs, and are committed to longstanding conflict resolution. This method requires a great deal of work, but it resolves conflicts successfully.

Resolution of Supervisor-Supervisee Conflict

Supervision is a knotty problem that can be exhilarating or taxing. There are resources to increase knowledge and skills in supervisors, but few to train supervisees. Good supervisory skills must be balanced with the skills of the supervisee. A leader cannot lead someone who refuses to follow. The success of supervision rests on both parties.

Supervision is a teaching and learning process. It is not a mechanism designed to share all positive or negative feedback. When a conflict arises in supervision, the following strategy may be useful:

1. Define the problem in action-oriented language. Be specific and try to limit the boundaries of the issue. It is more helpful to tell staff members to improve their telephone manners than to tell them that they must improve their attitude.
2. Share the feedback verbally and offer a written summary of the major points involved in the feedback. Defense mechanisms may distort the information that is shared.
3. Offer concrete examples of what was seen or heard. This helps to move unconscious reactions into conscious thoughts. For example, "The way that you took Mr. Collins' call was helpful, but Mrs. Edgar was angry because she was put on hold three times."
4. Use personal pronouns during the session. Tell the staff member that "I am angry because you . . . . " or "I liked the way that you handled . . . . " The use of *we* or *management* does not pinpoint the issues. Each party must admit to his or her own emotions and thoughts.
5. Express feelings, if possible, but try to concentrate on task-related concerns.
6. Offer several options to resolve the conflict by compromise or integration of differences.

Constructive Use of Small Group Conflict

Brill[27] viewed conflict as a constructive process and suggested the following process:

1. Accept the existence of conflict and view it as understandable, predictable, and manageable.
2. Create a climate in which differences among members are accepted. Allow free expression of feelings, thoughts, and emotions. Use other resources to deal with inappropriate feelings.
3. Define conflict. Identify sources, boundaries, and solutions.
4. Delineate areas of trust among members and expand the area of trust. An outsider may be helpful here.
5. Generate a list of alternatives. Select one solution.

A strategy for resolving small group conflict should be based on open communication, a delineation of the group's goals, a presentation of the conflict, and an opportunity to explore creative solutions. The steps of this strategy are

1. List the purpose and goals of the group.
2. Write a statement that indicates the nature of the conflict. Categorize the underlying causes of the conflict: resources, ideological, or personal identity. List the causes under each appropriate heading.
3. Allow a minimum of 30 minutes in which members express their feelings about the conflict. Encourage people to use personal pronouns such as *I* and *me*. The group should work to accept these expressions openly without comment. This ventilation period should help people to address emotional concerns and permit them to invest energy in the group task.
4. Move to conflict resolution. Members should write their ideas on a piece of paper. The ideas should be recopied so that all members can see all information.
5. Use compromise or integration to reach a resolution.

Cultural Aspects of Conflict Resolution

Conflicts emerge from differences among people, and differences are based on values. A value is an attitude, belief, or feeling that is learned. Family, peers, religious affiliates, and school personnel all shape values. People orient themselves to daily life by weighing input from the environment on an internal value scale. Values help people to function efficiently in the world, but they may become so automatic that they close a person's mind to new ideas or approaches to situations.

Values shape individual responses to confrontation and fighting. Some people are silent; some, aggressive; some, assertive; and some, active on selected issues. The group members must develop norms to handle decision making, fighting, and conflict in a positive manner.

ORGANIZATIONAL CONFLICT

Managers can assess organizational conflicts by using a theoretical model, since it frees them from the bias created by their own immediate involvement in the conflict. By analyzing conflict in a relatively objective manner, a manager can deal with it more positively and more easily. The following is a basic model for such an analysis:

1. The basic conflict
   a. Overt level
   b. The hidden agenda
   c. The source of conflict
2. The participants
   a. Immediate and primary participants
   b. Secondary participants
   c. The audience
3. The provision of an arena
4. The development of rules
5. Strategies for dealing with organizational conflict

Exhibit 17–3 is an example of the use of this model.

The Basic Conflict

Overt Level

As a starting point, the manager analyzing a conflict describes the obvious problem. This process of naming the conflict elements provides focus and clarifies the issues that are at stake. Examples include

- habitual lateness by an employee
- delays in transport of patients from inpatient service to physical therapy or occupation therapy service
- lack of clarity about job responsibilities
- delays in treating patients, causing patients to wait unduly for their appointments

The Hidden Agenda

While the overt issue may be the true and only substance of the conflict, there is sometimes another area of conflict that constitutes a hidden agenda. This hidden agenda item may be the true conflict, or it may be an adjunct issue. The process of naming the conflict and describing its elements helps bring to light any hidden agenda.

Conflict issues are buried for several reasons. They may be too explosive to deal with openly, or subconscious protective mechanisms may prevent a

Exhibit 17–3 Conflict Model with Example

The Basic Conflict	
Overt issue	Habitual lateness and/or absenteeism of employee
Hidden agenda	Growing employee resistance to managerial authority
Sources	Human need vs. organizational need Organizational structure
Participants	
Immediate	Unit supervisor and employee
Secondary	Chief of service, personnel director
Audience	Other employees with similar problem with work schedule, other managers with similar employee disciplinary problems, and higher levels of management who monitor organizational climate
Arena	Grievance procedure
Rules	Work rules re attendance, procedures for filing grievances
Strategy	Limitation of conflict to unit members

threatening subject from surfacing until the individual in question has a safe structure and the necessary support to deal with it. Within an institution, the climate may not be appropriate for accepting conflict, or organizational resources may be insufficient to deal with it.

The subtleties of intraorganizational power struggles cause certain aspects of conflict to remain hidden. Individuals may choose to obscure the real issue as a means of testing their strength, of determining points of opposition before plunging ahead with an issue, or of checking the intensity of opposition. Periodic sparring over issues that never seem to be resolved is a clue to the existence of a hidden agenda item. For example, the hospital budget issue of billing a medical group practice for certain administrative services may surface each year for temporary resolution. The root of the problem is not the allocation of money; it is the creation of a new institutional structure with organizational control of outpatient services at stake.

The Sources of Conflict

The definition of conflict provides the nucleus of its sources: the competition for resources, the authority relationships, the extraorganizational pressures. As discussed earlier, conflict has its source in the individuals who participate in organizational activities.

The Nature of the Organization. Organizations with multiple goals face competing and sometimes mutually exclusive demands for available resources. A hospital, for example, must safeguard against malpractice claims through active risk control management, yet it must contain costs. The rules, regulations, and requirements imposed by the many controllers of the organization identified in the clientele network may be a source of conflict. Shifting client demand and changes in the degree of client participation in the organization lead to conflict when an increase in the allocation of resources for one group is a loss for another. The authority structure is another clue to potential conflict; members of coercive organizations are more frequently in conflict with the organization than are members of normative institutions.

The Organizational Climate. An emphasis on competition as a means of enhancing productivity, as in the use of the "deadly parallel" pattern in organizational structure, or the use of a reward system that emphasizes competition among individuals or departments, as in sales and productivity, may cause conflict. The intentional overlap and blurred jurisdiction of units can produce continual jockeying for organizational territory. Competition for scarce resources may be sharp, with resulting conflict, coalitions, and compromises. The subtleties of an institution's power struggles, the shifting balance of power (e.g., the growing union movement), and the need to demonstrate power constitute another facet of organizational climate. Denial of conflict is a potential source of trouble, since it removes a safe outlet for resolution of conflict at its incipient level.

The Organizational Structure. The complex authority structure in health care organizations, i.e., a dual track of authority coupled with an increasing professionalism among the many specialized workers, creates situations of potential conflict. Professional practitioners, such as nurses, physical therapists, clinical psychologists, and social workers, are trained to assess patient needs and to take actions within the scope of licensure or certification; however, their ability to make decisions is limited by the hierarchical organizational structure. This problem is compounded when the individual practitioner has a legal duty to act or refrain from acting that is directly opposite to the hierarchical system, such as when a nurse refrains from giving a medication that would be harmful to the patient even when the physician has (inadvertently) ordered such a dosage.

Physicians, in holding staff appointments, find themselves required to shift regularly from their roles as independent practitioners when functioning outside the health care facility to more limited roles as members of the organizational hierarchy. This regular role shift may also be required of the physical therapist, nurse-practitioner, or occupational therapist who functions as an independent agent in private practice and at the same time participates in the patient care process as a staff member of a health care institution.

Conflict may also arise from specialization within the organizational structure when all individuals attempt to carry out their own assigned activity. For example, the social worker seeks to place a patient in a long-term care facility, but the utilization review coordinator must impose strict guidelines in terms of days of care allotted under certain payment contracts. The medical record practitioner must develop a system of record control, although many users of the record find it more practical to retain records in restricted areas of their own. The purchasing agent must comply with certain regulations on deadlines, budget restrictions, and auditing procedures in spite of individual needs. Specialization within the complexities of bureaucratization leads to frustration, misunderstanding, and, thus, conflict.

The aspect of superior-subordinate relationships constitutes another area of potential conflict. The organization chart is, in fact, a suppression chart that specifies which positions have authority over and literally suppress other individual jobs or units. The legitimacy of leaders' claim to office is continually assessed. The power, prestige, and rewards built into the hierarchical system all represent gain for some and related loss for others. The erosion of traditional territory associated with line management results from activity clearly intended to remove some authority from the line manager. These include client or worker involvement in decision making.

The process of management by objectives in which the worker is directly involved in setting and assessing objectives commands much attention for its motivational value. Streamlined processes, such as central number assignments or patient bed assignments, have much merit as systems improvements; a central pool of patient aides, assistants, and transporters is an alternative to assignment by department. Yet each of these processes erodes the distinct territory of one or several managers, whose ability to make decisions is affected by such systems changes. Increased specialization in some technical areas leads to a more frequent use of functional specialists. Although the line manager retains authority, the specialist must be included in the planning and decision-making process; the line manager is no longer the sole agent.

Unions may invade managerial territory in several areas relating to personnel management and direct work assignment. In the collective bargaining process, what work, who will do it, and how much will be done may be issues. Union gains may be management losses.

Individual vs. Organizational Needs. Human needs and values must be welded into the organizational framework. A large number of clients and workers enter the organization, and they have different values, experience, motives, and expectations. The degree to which each individual internalizes the values of the organization and accepts a primary identity derived from the institution varies greatly. Individuals who do not participate directly in the accomplishment of organizational goals or in the institutional authority structure tend to have less identification with the establishment and view its demands differently from those who participate more fully in direct, goal-oriented activities.

Solutions to Previous Conflicts. New problems may arise from solutions to previous conflicts. The use of compromise as a strategy in dealing with conflict tends to leave all participants somewhat dissatisfied. At the next opportunity, one or more participants may seek to reopen the issue in order to regain what was lost, particularly if the loss was acute. The loser may build up resources and enter into an active state of aggression when such resources have been accumulated, such as a nation defeated after a war (e.g., Germany after World War I). When there is a consistent denial pattern, the conflict may "go underground" for a time, then emerge again with greater force. Again, managers should realistically examine the negative consequences of conflict resolutions in order to minimize their recurrence.

The Participants

The immediate participants in the conflict can be identified readily as the individuals or groups caught in the open exchange. The secondary participants are the individuals called in to take an active role, such as persons in the next level of the hierarchy. A manager may consult with a senior official to whom the individual involved in the conflict reports or with a staff adviser, such as a labor relations specialist. A unit manager may be required in some instances to refer conflict to the next level for resolution, as in some grievance procedures. In the case of a unionized employee, a representative of the union, such as a shop steward, may be involved. A "neutral" may be called in by both parties in a labor dispute, e.g., a mediator or an arbitrator. Occasionally, a manager may consult informally with certain "marginal" individuals, such as those in the department or organization who have an overlapping role set, a supervisor whose domain spans several activities, a client who is also on an advisory committee, or another department head who has faced similar situations. Because they link groups, these individuals are sought out in order to test a potential solution or to obtain information and even advice.

A third category of participants may be classified as the audience. This category may include

- the clients. If the conflict is overt and severe, clients may turn to other organizations for the necessary services in order to avoid the conflict. On the other hand, uncertainty may cause tension within this group, and clients may become active participants. A client group alientated from the institution may develop its own system to meet its needs.

- the public at large. This group may seek action through recourse to some government agency and an agency's intervention into the conflict may take the form of additional regulation of the organization. The conflict may be brought into the public arena; for example, a labor dispute may be taken to court. The net effect of intervention by some agent on behalf of the public at large is the opening or broadening of the conflict, which removes it from the immediate control of the original parties to the dispute.

- a potential rival or enemy. While one group and its opponents are absorbed in conflict, a third group whose energies are not drained by conflict may seek to expand its services and attract the clients of the groups locked in the dispute.

- individuals or groups with similar complaints. Some observers may seek to press a similar claim if "the right side" wins. In the case of employee unrest, a labor organizer may consider more active unionization attempts. Independent practitioners who seek greater autonomy in the practice of health care may monitor changes in organizational bylaws or state licensure regulations and find gains made by one individual or group of practitioners the catalyst needed to obtain a similar gain. In malpractice cases, jury awards are monitored and publicized; as the basis for such claims is expanded through trends in court decisions, more individuals may advance their cases when, without such publicity in the benchmark cases, this basis of claim might not have arisen. A worker who sees another worker win a concession from the manager about some work rule will more readily press a similar claim.

- the opportunist. Some individual or group may seek to enter the conflict as champion or savior. Such action may be undertaken by individuals seeking to raise themselves to leadership positions.

In many cases, the audience not only cheers and jeers, but also becomes active participants, thus expanding the conflict in terms of the number of individuals or groups who must be satisfied in any solution.

Conflict should be resolved at as low an organizational level as possible. The facts are better known by the immediate participants, and face-to-face, immediate communication is possible. Because the number of participants is limited, agreement to the solution may be more easily obtained. Top levels of management should be involved only rarely in conflicts within the organization, because their involvement might give undue weight or proportion to the problem, establish precedent, and force the setting of policy that escalates resolutions to a higher level. The resources of top management generally are reserved for critical issues.

The Provision of an Arena

The development of a safe, predictable, accessible arena tends to create a sense of security and to keep the problems from becoming diffuse. The aggrieved know where to turn and what to do in order to seek redress. The provision of an acceptable arena is also efficient. The individuals involved give their attention to it in a highly structured manner, and it establishes clear boundaries to the conflict. It is legitimate to bring issues of conflict to this place, through this structure, at these designated times. The court system and legislative debate are such arenas in the larger society. In organizations, arenas include the structured grievance process for employees (Exhibit 17–4), the appeals process for the professional staff member seeking staff appointment, or the complaint department for customers. Committees in which multiple input is invited are also common arenas that have been developed in organizational settings.

Exhibit 17–4 Excerpts from Grievance Procedure

Any grievance which may arise between the parties concerning the application, meaning, or interpretation of this Agreement shall be resolved in the following manner:

Step 1: An employee having a grievance and his Union delegate shall discuss it with his immediate supervisor within five (5) working days after it arose or should have been made known to the employee. The Hospital shall give its response through the supervisor to the employee and to this Union delegate within five (5) working days after the presentation of the grievance. In the event no appeal is taken to the next step (Step 2) the decision rendered in this step shall be final.

Step 2: If the grievance is not settled in Step 1, the grievance may, within five (5) working days after the answer in Step 1, be presented in Step 2. When grievances are presented in Step 2, they shall be reduced to writing on grievance forms provided by the Hospital (which shall then be assigned a number by the Personnel Services at the Union's request), signed by the grievant and his Union representative, and presented to the Department Head and the Department of Personnel Services. A grievance so presented in Step 2 shall be answered in writing within five (5) working days after its presentation.

The Development of Rules

Rules serve to limit the energy expended on the conflict process. The provision of rules has a face-saving and legitimizing effect; it is permissible to disagree, equal time is guaranteed, and each point of view is aired. The rules also provide a basis for the intervention of a referee or neutral. The rules may be developed to allow a cooling-off period so that the issues can be put in perspective. The time frame given by the rules reduces uneasiness, since participants are assured of a legitimate opportunity to present the issues. Conflict remains under control.

Strategies for Dealing with Organizational Conflict

Two strategies for dealing with conflict are opposite approaches: limitation and purposeful expansion. The limitation of conflict as a strategy was developed by E.E. Schattschneider, who noted the contagiousness of conflict. An organization runs the risk of losing control as conflict is widened, and it is unlikely that both sides will be reinforced equally. Conflict is best kept private, limited, and therefore controllable.[29]

An underlying purpose of the intentional expansion of conflict is to demonstrate its immediate effect on the clients or the public, who in turn will bring pressure on the opposing party to end the dispute. The immediate involvement of the client group is sought in the hope that it will act as a catalytic factor, forcing quick resolution. For example, a teachers' union may go on strike at the beginning of a school year, a coal miners' union may strike during the winter high fuel consumption season, traffic officers may conduct a slowdown or job action during the height of the Fourth of July traffic to the shore.

The routinization of conflict is a third strategy. Another aspect of this strategy may be seen in the symbolic value of the short strike that is a kind of catharsis, an annual or biennial event. Other strategies include concepts noted in other discussions, e.g., cooptation, strategic leniency, preformed decisions, and the selection of individuals who fit the organization.

In addition to such conscious strategy, a manager has the general principles of sound organization. When used properly, these principles bring about stability and reduce conflict. Known policies and rules, sufficient orientation and training of members, proper authority-responsibility designations, and clear chain of command and communication: these practices foster cooperation and mutual expectation, with the attendant reduction of undue conflict.

NOTES

1. G.A. Kimble and N. Garmezy, *Principles of General Psychology* (New York: Ronald Press, 1962), p. 485.

2. C.S. Hall, *A Primer of Freudian Psychology* (New York: Mentor, 1954), p. 121.

3. C.S. Hall and V.J. Nordby, *A Primer of Jungian Psychology* (New York: Mentor, 1972), p. 69.

4. Erik H. Erikson, "Eight Ages of Man," in *Readings in Child Behavior and Development,* ed. C.S. Lavatelli and F. Stendler (New York: Harcourt, 1972), pp. 19–30.

5. C.S. Hall and G. Lindzey, *Theories of Personality* (New York: John Wiley, 1957), p. 442.

6. Ibid., p. 428.

7. Ibid., p. 424.

8. Neal E. Miller, *Neal E. Miller: Selected Papers on Conflict, Displacement, Learned Drives & Theory* (Chicago: Aldine-Atherton, 1971), p. 67.

9. Kimble and Garmezy, *Principles of General Psychology,* p. 485.

10. Ibid., p. 486.

11. Ibid.

12. Ibid., p. 487.

13. Ibid., p. 505.

14. Ibid.

15. Kurt Lewin, *A Dynamic Theory of Personality,* trans. D.K. Adams and K. Zener (New York: McGraw-Hill, 1935).

16. Kurt Lewin, *Resolving Social Conflicts* (New York: Harper & Row, 1948).

17. E.E. Sampson and M.S. Martas, *Group Process for the Health Professional* (New York: John Wiley, 1977), p. 22.

18. W.R. Bion, *Experiences in Groups* (New York: Basic Books, 1959), pp. 59–60.

19. M.S. Olmstead, *The Small Group* (New York: Random House, 1959), pp. 20–22.

20. R.W. Napier and M.K. Gershenfield, *Groups: Theory & Experience* (Boston: Houghton-Mifflin, 1973), pp. 24–27.

21. M.J. Rioch, "All We Like Sheep . . . [Isaiah 53:6]: Followers and Leaders," *Psychiatry* 34 (1971): 258–273.

22. N.I. Brill, *Teamwork* (Philadelphia: J.B. Lippincott, 1976), pp. 72–74.

23. W.C. Schutz, *Firo: A Three-Dimensional Theory of Interpersonal Behavior* (New York: Holt, 1958).

24. Bion, *Experiences in Groups.*

25. B.W. Tuchman, "Developmental Sequence in Small Groups," *Psychological Bulletin* 63 (1965): 384–399.

26. Ibid.

27. Brill, ibid.

28. R. Goldhammer, *Clinical Supervision* (New York: Holt, Rinehart & Winston, 1969), p. 83.

29. E.E. Schattschneider, *The Semisovereign People* (New York: Holt, Rinehart & Winston, 1960), pp. 1–18.

Conclusion

This work began with a discussion of the traditional functions of the manager. What qualifies an individual to assume the role of manager? As with the grant of organizational authority, the first pillar is the manager's technical and professional ability. In the health care setting, department heads and chiefs of service are specialists, usually trained in a specific health care discipline, such as nursing, physical therapy, occupational therapy, medical technology, or health records administration. Education for specific health disciplines usually includes some training in management techniques, but this is not the primary focus.

What, then, is the suggested plan of action for the health care practitioner who assumes a greater, more specific management role? What program of study and activity will equip the manager to deal with conflict, change, shifting balances of power, and authority? How does the manager avoid the extremes of "bureausis" and "bureaupathology"? Education is the answer. Managers must seek to increase their skills in the management area through formal study. This program of study should go beyond specific technical and professional skills (e.g., cost accounting in budget preparation) to embrace a wide range of social science areas. Psychology and sociology provide insights into interpersonal relationships; history and political science, into change in the social and political culture.

Managers must develop the capacity for balance and inner harmony that characterizes the whole person. They turn to music, art, philosophy, and related disciplines to enrich their own spirits, mindful of the Greek aphorism: "One becomes similar to what one contemplates." The work of health care, with its long history of compassionate involvement with the ill and infirm, demands much from the health care practitioner who must balance the science of management with the art of human relations.

Index

A

Acceptance, zone of, 137, 140-141, 143, 144
Acceptance or consent theory of formal authority, 137-138
Accessibility, 47
Account codes, 225-226
Accreditation, 293. *See also* Joint Commission on the Accreditation of Hospitals
Accuracy, 32, 207
Acoustics, 47
Action, 41, 102
Activities
  definition of, 181, 203
  as phase of PERT network, 182-186
  real, 185-186
  specification sheet for, 186-187
Adaptation strategy, 297-298
Adjustments, salary, 236
Administrative Management Society, 196
Administrative systems, 11
Advisers, 52, 283
Age Discrimination in Employment Act, 26
Alignment charts, 208-210
Ambivalent pattern, 129
American Association of Blood Banks, 293
American Association of Hospital Accountants, 225

American Civil Liberties Union, 282
American Hospital Association, 28, 224, 232, 283
American Medical Association, 283
American Medical Record Association, 29-30, 283
American Occupational Therapy Association, 29
American Osteopathic Association, 277
American Physical Therapy Association, 29
American Psychiatric Association, 293
American Red Cross, 293, 298-299
American Society of Mechanical Engineers, 196
Appeal procedure, 155
Approval process, 229-230
Archetypes, 165
Architects, 46, 48-50
Argyris, Chris, 9
Authoritarian leadership, 146
Authority, 133-159
  acceptance of, 138, 140-141
  coercive, 75, 270
  delineation of, 99-100, 136, 140
  formal, 135-140
  functional, 141-142
  rational-legal, 139, 270, 274
  restrictions on, 74, 100, 143-144
  sources of, 137-143
  types of, 74, 138-139, 270
  views of, 128-129, 138
  See also Power

R

Random condition, 207
Random number tables, 213-214,
  215-216
Rationalization, 326
Reactions, anticipated, 138
Records, federal regulation of, 284
"Red tape," 60, 273, 274
Regional Comprehensive Health
  Planning programs, 306
Regional Medical Programs, 306
Regulations, 25, 26, 45-50
Remedial actions. *See* Deviations,
  correction of
Reports, 55, 121-122
Repression, 326
Reprimand, written, 123
Research, 64-65, 84-85, 272, 299
Resource suppliers, 280-281
Responsibility centers, 227
Results management. *See* Management
  by Objectives
Revenues, 224, 230
Review process, budgetary, 229-230
Rhocrematics, 11
Rites, 126
Rodriguez, Arthur A. and Alfred
  Rodriguez, 239-241
Roethlisberger, F.J., 8
Role playing, 157
Root and branch decisions, 56-57
Rotating shifts, 123
Rules, 41, 120, 274
Rumors, 168

S

Sampling. *See* Work sampling
Sanctions, 123
Satisficing, 57
Scalar principle, 73
Schattschneider, E.E., 337
Scheduling charts, 174-176
Schlesinger, Leonard, 308

Schutz, W.C., 324
Scientific management, 8
Scientists, 10
Scott, W. Richard, 269-270, 273
Self-discipline, 153
Self-motivation, 130, 147, 250
Selznick, Philip, 294
Seminars, 157
Services, fee for, 241-244
Short interval scheduling, 15
Sill, David, 298
Simon, Herbert, 51, 137-138
Simulation (model building), 65
Situation, law of the, 141-142
Social distance, 163
Social reform, 299
Society, influences of, 140, 163
Space, uses of, 168
Specialization, 72, 268, 273, 303,
  333
Staff
  assignment of, 4
  assistance of, on committees, 105
  authority, 97, 141
  medical, 53, 79, 80
  See also Line and staff function;
    Personnel
Standards, 172, 173
Standing committees, 97, 108
Statistical principles, 206-207
Status concerns, 169
Step budget, 224
Stochastic simulation, 65-66
Storage, 197
Strikes, labor, 314-315
Structuralism, 9
Subgoals. *See* Events
Subjective, Objective, Assessment
  Plan (SOAP), 156
Subnetworks, 186
Subordinates, 137-138
Subsidiary plans, 223
Succession, pattern of, 139
Summary task list, 203
Supervision, 133-159. *See also*
  Management

About the Authors

JOAN GRATTO LIEBLER, R.R.A, M.P.A., is Professor in the Department of Health Records Administration, College of Allied Health Professions, Temple University. She is responsible for the management sequence of the curriculum. In addition to working in a variety of health care settings, Mrs. Liebler has taught a variety of workshops in the areas of applied management practice. She is on the editorial boards of *Topics in Medical Record Administration* and *Health Care Supervisor,* quarterly publications of Aspen Systems Corporation. She is a member of the American Medical Record Association and has held office at the state and national level.

RUTH ELLEN LEVINE, ED.D., O.T.R., is Professor and Chairman of the Department of Occupational Therapy, College of Allied Health Sciences, Thomas Jefferson University. She received her education at the University of Pennsylvania and Temple University. Levine founded a homecare private practice group in 1974 and served as president of the group until 1983. She has also contributed to several textbooks and journals.

HYMAN LEO DERVITZ, L.P.T., M.A., is Professor and Chairman of the Department of Physical Therapy, College of Allied Health Professions, Temple University. He was formerly director of a large physical therapy department in a rehabilitation hospital. He has lectured extensively on the topic of health care management in the academic setting and at professional meetings. He is co-editor of the *Handbook for Physical Therapy Teachers* and has written numerous articles for professional journals. He is a member of the American Physical Therapy Association and has served as President of a state chapter and as member of the Board of Directors on the national level.